Instructor's Manual

SPORTS INJURY MANAGEMENT

Instructor's Manual

Prepared by:

Malissa Martin, Ph.D., A.T.,C.
Director, Athletic Training Curriculum Program
Department of Physical Education
University of South Carolina
Columbia, South Carolina

To Accompany the First Edition of:

SPORTS INJURY MANAGEMENT

Marcia K. Anderson, Ph.D., L.A.T.,C.
Professor and Director, Athletic Training Curriculum Program
Department of Movement Arts, Health Promotions, and Leisure Studies
Bridgewater State College
Bridgewater, Massachusetts

Susan J. Hall, Ph.D.
Professor and Director of Graduate Studies
Department of Kinesiology and Physical Education
California State University, Northridge
Northridge, California

SANS TACHE

Williams & Wilkins
BALTIMORE • PHILADELPHIA • HONG KONG
LONDON • MUNICH • SYDNEY • TOKYO
A WAVERLY COMPANY

1995

Executive Editor: Donna Balado
Developmental Editor: Victoria Vaughn
Production Coordinator: Peter J. Carley
Project Editor: Arlene Sheir-Allen

Rose Tree Corporate Center
1400 North Providence Road
Building II, Suite 5025
Media, PA 19063-2043 USA

Accurate indications, adverse reactions, and dosage schedules for drugs are provided in this book, but it is possible they may change. The reader is urged to review the package information data of the manufacturers of the medications mentioned.

Printed in the United States of America

The Publishers have made every effort to trace the copyright holders for borrowed material. If they have inadvertently overlooked any, they will be pleased to make the necessary arrangements at the first opportunity.

95 96 97 98 99
1 2 3 4 5 6 7 8 9 10

Preface

This Instructor's Manual was written specifically for the first edition of *Sports Injury Management.* The purpose of this manual is to provide the instructor with useful exercises, experiences, and teaching strategies to reinforce and enhance the concepts and material presented in the text. The manual provides the instructor and student with an active learning, problem solving and critical thinking approach to situations involved in athletic training and athletic health care.

Designed to correspond with the chapters of the text, chapters in this manual include:

Learning Objectives … pinpoints important student learning goals

Anatomy Review … provides for a review of anatomical structures associated with the chapter

Key Terminology … stresses important terms and their meaning

Kinematics … provides for range of motion, muscle action, and function measurements

Simulations … provides for critical thinking exercises through the use of injury scenarios, leading the student from one part of a scenario to the next. Many of the scenarios parallel those presented in the text and Student Manual

Situations … provides for critical thinking exercises associated with specific athletic injury situations

Teaching Strategies … provides for additional exercises to be used as teaching strategies

Chapter Test Questions … multiple choice questions for students or as additional resources for examination questions

A special thanks to: Marcia Anderson for asking me to write the instructor's materials for *Sports Injury Management* and giving me an opportunity for another learning experience; Andy Bosman for his time and patience in doing the desktop publishing for the manual; Nikki Lukas for her efforts in editing the manual; Kim Shibinski, who has given me the support and encouragement to continue to reach for my dreams and accomplish my goals; and Carol Lugge, who opened my door into the world of teaching and academia.

Malissa Martin

CONTENTS

Chapter 1 Sports Injury Management and the Athletic Trainer

<u>After completing this chapter the student should be able to:</u>

- **Identify health care services in sports medicine that enhance health fitness and sport performance.**
- **Identify members of the primary sports medicine team, their role and responsibility in sport injury management.**
- **Explain basic parameters of ethical conduct and standards of professional practice for athletic trainers.**
- **Specify academic and clinical requirements necessary to become a National Athletic Trainers' Association (NATA) certified athletic trainer, and continuing education requirements needed to maintain certification.**
- **Explain standard of care of what factors must be proved to show breach of duty of care.**
- **Describe preventative measures to reduce potential risk of litigation.**
- **Discuss potential job opportunities for an individual interested in athletic training as a career option.**

I. Key Terms

<u>Instructions</u>: *Instruct the students to define the following terms.*

Sports medicine
Standard of care
Informed consent
Negligence
Gross negligence
Tort
Battery
Foreseeability of harm
Malfeasance
Misfeasance
Nonfeasance
Malpractice
Implied warranty
Expressed warranty
Modalities

II. Simulations

Instructions: *Divide the students into groups and have them exchange roles from simulation to simulation as they perform the following simulated experiences.*

1 **You have learned that several high school athletes are using the weight room when a supervisor is not present. Although the athletes have been instructed in proper lifting technique and safety, you are concerned about legal liability. What implications exist concerning your legal responsibility to these athletes?**

1A. What actions should be taken to ensure a safe weight room facility?

2 **You are a college athletic trainer, and you have a student who wants to pursue NATA certification. There is no accredited curriculum program at your college. How will you guide and help this student in his/her pursuit?**

2A. The student has successfully passed the NATA certification examination and is now a certified athletic trainer. What type of continuing education requirements must the student know?

III. Situations

Instructions: *Have each student work with a partner to cooperatively analyze and answer the following situations.*

1. You have just been named the athletic trainer at a major high school. You are the first athletic trainer in the history of the high school and must develop a sports medicine team. What individuals might you have on your team?

2. You are a high school athletic trainer and have just been asked by your athletic director to justify your position at the school to the school board. How would you do this?

3. An athlete sustains an injury. What standards of care and professional conduct should the athlete expect from an immediate health care provider?

III. Situations (Con't)

4. A soccer player received a severe blow to the anterior right thigh that resulted in rapid swelling. The athletic trainer applied ice to limit swelling and referred the athlete to a physician. The athlete decided not to see the physician and returned home to ice the leg. Three days later the swelling was still present, and the soccer player had problems moving the foot of the injured leg. If litigation occurred as a result of this injury what should the athletic trainer have done to protect against possible legal action?

IV. Teaching Strategies

1. Invite a lawyer to class to discuss the legal ramifications associated with standards of care for athletic trainers.

2. Develop a panel composed of a team physician, primary care physician, athletic trainer, and physical therapist. Have them discuss their role in the sports medicine team.

3. Invite an athletic director to class to discus the role and duties of the athletic trainer from an administrator's point of view.

4. Have students develop their own informed consent forms, medical history forms, and injury report forms for a high school or college athletic setting.

5. Divide students into groups and have them develop a full preseason medical examination for a team or group of athletes. Have the student include stations, medical personnel, equipment facilities, and forms needed for the examination.

Instructor's Key

I. Key Terms

Sports medicine	Area of health and special services that apply medical and scientific knowledge to prevent, recognize, manage, and rehabilitate injuries related to sport, exercise, and/or recreational activity.
Standard of care	What action another minimally competent professional educated and practicing in the same profession would have taken in the same or similar circumstance to protect an individual from harm.
Informed consent	Condition whereby an injured adult, or parents of minor children, has been reasonably informed of needed treatment, possible alternative treatments, and advantages and disadvantages of each course of action, and gives written consent to receive treatment.
Negligence	Breach of one's duty of care that causes harm to another individual.
Gross negligence	Breach of one's duty of care that causes harm to another individual.
Tort	A wrong done to an individual whereby the injured party seeks a remedy for damages suffered.
Battery	Unpermitted or intentional contact with another individual without their consent.
Foreseeability of harm	Condition whereby danger is apparent, or should have been apparent, resulting in an unreasonably unsafe condition.
Malfeasance	Committing an act that is not your responsibility to perform.
Misfeasance	Committing an act that is your responsibility to perform, but the wrong procedure is followed, or the right procedure is done in an improper manner.
Nonfeasance	Failing to perform one's legal duty of care.
Malpractice	Committing a negligent act while providing care.

Implied warranty — — — Unwritten guarantee that the product is reasonably safe when used for its intended purpose.

Expressed warranty — — Written guarantee that states the product is safe for consumer use.

Modalities — — — — — — — Therapeutic agents that enhance tissue healing while reducing pain and disability.

II. Simulations

1

Did the students determine that their duty of care is relative to the athletes lifting weights in an unsupervised weight room? Did they take the following course of action:

- foresee the possibility of injury
- warn the individuals to leave the weight room
- take immediate action to close the weight room until competent personnel could supervise the area.

Failure to perform these actions could make the athletic trainer liable through the act of nonfeasance.

1A. Did the students' preventive measures include:

- posting signs that no one is allowed in the weight room unless supervised by competent personnel
- posting signs on the walls of the weight room depicting proper lifting techniques for each lift
- locking the weight room when there is no supervisor

2 NATA certification and continuing education requirements

Did the students determine that the following need to be accomplished prior to the individual becoming a certified athletic trainer?

- the completion of formal instruction in anatomy/physiology, kinesiology/biomechanics, exercise physiology, basic athletic training, and advanced athletic training.
- 1500 clinical hours under the direct supervision of a certified athletic trainer
- proof of graduation at the baccalaureate level at an accredited college or university
- at least 25% of clinical athletic training experiences must be attained in practice and/or game coverage with one or more of the following sports: football, soccer, wrestling, gymnastics, hockey, wrestling, basketball, lacrosse, volleyball, and rugby
- endorsement by a certified athletic trainer
- current CPR certification
- success in passing the NATA examination

2A. Did the students determine that after an individual becomes certified that individual must meet the following continuing education requirements to maintain certification:

- eight continuing education units over a three-year period
- current proof of CPR certification at least once during the three-year period

Refer to pages 13-14 in the text.

III. Situations

1. **Sports Medicine Team** - Did the students' sports medicine team include:
   - team physician
   - athletic trainer
   - primary care physician
   - other professional health personnel

   Refer to Table 1-1 on page 6 in the text.

2. **Duties of the Athletic Trainer** - Did the students include the following duties to justify their position as an athletic trainer?
   - injury prevention
   - recognition and evaluation of injuries/illnesses
   - injury management/treatment and disposition
   - injury rehabilitation
   - organization and administration of athletic health care
   - education and counseling of athletes

   Refer to Table 1-2 on page 9 in text.

III. Situations (Con't)

3. Standard of Professional Practice - Did the students determine that the individual providing the care should be an NATA certified athletic trainer and that the standard of care should reflect the profession of athletic training?

4. Injury Report - In administering care to the injured soccer player, did the students determine that an injury report should be completed documenting the injury and the need to see a physician?

Refer to Field Strategy 1-7 on page 28 in the text.

Chapter 2 The Mechanics of Tissue Injury and Healing

After completing this chapter the student should be able to:

- **Define compression, tension, shear, stress, strain, bending, and torsion and explain how each can play a role in injury to biological tissue**
- **Explain how the material constituent and structural organization of skin, tendon, ligament, muscle, and bone affect the ability of these structures to withstand the mechanical loads to which each is subjected**
- **List and describe common injuries of skin, tendons, ligaments, muscles, and bone**
- **Describe the processes by which nerves are injured and the processes by which nerves can heal**
- **Discuss the types of altered sensation that can result from nerve injury**

I. Key Terms

Instructions: *Instruct the students to define the following terms.*

Torsion
Bending
Yield point
Anisotropic
Viscoelastic
Zone of primary injury
Zone of secondary injury
Cancellous
Cortical
Chemosensitive
Mechanosensitive
Phagocytosis
Edema
Ecchymosis
Adhesions
Stress
Osteopenia
Failure
Fracture
Stress fracture
Callus
Cramp
Spasm
Contusion
Myositis
Myositis ossificans
Hematoma
Strain
Tendinitis
Tenosynovitis
Calcific tendinitis
Bursitis
Fascitis
Hypoxia
Necrosis
Dermatome
Afferent nerves
Efferent nerves
Nociceptors
Neuroma
Neurotmesis
Amenorrhea

II. Simulations

Instructions: *Divide the students into groups of three with one student being the injured athlete, another the athletic trainer, and the third student an observer. Have the students exchange roles from simulation to simulation as they perform the following simulated experiences.*

1 **A runner reports to you with localized shin pain that has been increasingly bothersome for a few weeks. What type of injury/injuries might you suspect?**

1A. Since the runner's pain has been present for a few weeks, it probably is a chronic or stress injury. In reference to the runner's training, what suggestions can you give to reduce the incidence of this injury recurring?

2 **A baseball player was hit in the thigh by a wild pitch while batting. What injuries should be suspected? If the injury is superficial, what signs and symptoms might you suspect?**

2A. After noting the signs and symptoms associated with a superficial contusion, demonstrate how to determine the severity of this injury.

3 **A weight lifter complains of pain radiating down the posterior aspect of the leg along with hypesthesia. What condition might you suspect and why?**

3A. Knowing that radiating pain and hypesthesia might indicate nerve involvement, describe the treatment protocol for this injury?

III. Situations

Instructions: *Have each student work with a partner to cooperatively analyze and answer the following situations.*

1. A running back was sandwiched between two players while being tackled. As a result, the running back sustained a thigh contusion. What type of load and force was associated with this injury?

2. A rugby player's leg is anchored to the ground and is tackled on that leg from the front while being pushed into the tackle from behind. A bending moment is created on the lower leg. What type of injury do you suspect to occur to the lower leg?

3. An athlete approaches you and questions why he/she has been told to do static stretching for a period of 30 seconds for each stretch rather than doing short ballistic stretches. How would you address this question?

4. A basketball player has sustained an ankle injury. Describe degrees of injury including crepitus, tissue damage, and signs and symptoms.

5. An athlete reports to you complaining of pain over the big toe. The athlete reports no recollection of injury. How would you determine if the toe is inflamed?

6. An adolescent athlete has sustained a routine ankle sprain. The pain continues to be localized at the joint line. After 2 weeks of conservative treatment, there is little to no improvement in the signs or symptoms of the injury. What type of injury should be suspected and why?

7. A sedentary 60-year-old woman wants to begin a weight-bearing exercise program. What precautions should be taken to prevent a bone injury? Why?

IV. Teaching Strategies

1. **Invite a radiologist to class to demonstrate the various types of diagnostic tools used to evaluate soft tissue injuries. Also have the radiologist demonstrate various types of fractures seen through radiographs.**

2. **Invite a pediatrician to class to further discuss pathological differences in bone injuries to immature and mature bones.**

3. **Take a field trip to a nearby medical facility or hospital to observe how x-ray and other diagnostic tools such as MRI and CT-scans are performed.**

Instructor's Key

I. Key Terms

Torsion	Twisting around an object's longitudinal axis in response to an applied torque
Bending	Loading that produces tension on one side of an object and compression on the other side
Yield point	The maximum load that a material can sustain without permanent deformation
Anisotropic	Having different strengths in response to loads from different directions
Viscoelastic	Responding to loading over time with changing rates of deformation
Zone of primary injury	Region of injured tissue prior to vasodilation
Zone of secondary injury	Region of damaged tissue following vasodilation
Cancellous	Bone tissue of relatively low density
Cortical	Compact bone tissue of relatively high density
Chemosensitive	Sensitive to chemical stimulation
Mechanosensitive	Sensitive to mechanical stimulation
Phagocytosis	Process by which white blood cells surround and digest foreign particles
Edema	Swelling resulting from collection of exuded lymph fluid in the interstitial tissues
Ecchymosis	Superficial tissue discoloration
Adhesions	Tissues that bind the healing tissue to adjacent structures, such as other ligaments or bone
Stress	The distribution of force within a body; quantified as force divided by the area over which the force acts

I. Key Terms (Con't)

Osteopenia	Condition of reduced bone mineral density that predisposes the individual to fractures
Failure	Loss of continuity; rupture of soft tissue or fracture of the bone
Fracture	A disruption in the continuity of a bone
Stress fracture	Fracture resulting from repeated loading with relatively low magnitude of force
Callus	Fibrous tissue containing immature bone tissue that forms at fracture sites during repair and regeneration
Cramp	Painful involuntary muscle contraction, either clonic or tonic
Spasm	Transitory muscle contractions
Contusion	Compression injury involving accumulation of blood and lymph within a muscle
Myositis	Inflammation of connective tissue within a muscle
Myositis ossificans	Accumulation of mineral deposits in a muscle
Hematoma	A localized mass of blood and lymph confined within a space or tissue
Strain	Amount of deformation with respect to the original dimensions of the structure
Tendinitis	Inflammation of a tendon
Tenosynovitis	Inflammation of a tendon sheath
Calcific tendinitis	Accumulation of mineral deposits in a tendon
Bursitis	Inflammation of a bursa
Fascitis	Inflammation of the fascia surrounding portions of a muscle
Hypoxia	Having a reduced concentration of oxygen
Necrosis	Death of a tissue

Key Terms (Con't)

Dermatome ———— A region of the skin supplied by a single afferent neuron

Afferent nerves ———— Nerves carrying sensory input from receptors in the skin, muscles, tendons, and ligaments to the central nervous system

Efferent nerves —————— Nerves carrying stimuli from the central nervous system to the muscles

Nociceptors ————— Specialized nerve endings that transduce pain

Neuroma ———————— A nerve tumor

Neurotmesis ————— Complete severance of a nerve

Amenorrhea ——————— Condition involving cessation of menses

II. Simulations

1 Chronic Injury

Did the students suspect the runner's injury was a chronic or stress injury?

1A. To decrease the recurrence of this injury, did the students suggest progression of intensity, change in running surface, and change in shoes during conditioning sessions?

2 Superficial Contusion

Did the students suspect the baseball player had a contusion? Did they note that ecchymosis may be present if the hemorrhage is superficial?

2A. To determine the severity of the contusion, did the students have the injured athlete perform knee range of motion to note limitations in movement?

3 Nerve Injury

Because of the radiating pain, did the students identify that the weight lifter may be experiencing some sort of nerve injury?

3A. Did the students' treatment plan include medical referral?

III. Situations

1. Axial Load - Did the students determine that an axial load and compression force were associated with the thigh contusion of the running back?

2. Lower Leg Fracture - Did the students determine what may have occurred when a tension force was applied to the leg of the rugby player? Since a bone can resist compression forces much better than tension forces, did they identify that a possible fracture may have occurred?

3. Stretching - Did the students determine that because of the viscoelastic aspect of muscle extensibility, it enables the muscle to stretch to greater lengths over time in response to a sustained tensile force? A static stretch maintained over a period of 30 seconds is more effective in increasing muscle length than a series of short ballistic stretches.

4. Ankle Injury - Did the students look for the following signs and symptoms to determine the degree of injury to the basketball player's ankle?

-degree of discomfort and pain
-local tenderness
-degree of swelling
-ecchymosis
-function

5. Inflammation - Did the students determine that inflammation of the big toe would exhibit the following signs and symptoms?

-redness (rubor)
-local heat (calor)
-swelling (tumor)
-pain (dolor)
-loss of function (function laesa)

6. Epiphyseal Injury - Did the students suspect an ankle epiphyseal injury in the adolescent athlete? Did they derive this conclusion based on the age of the athlete and the lack of improvement of the injury after conservative treatment?

7. Senior Athlete - Did the students suggest that the 60-year-old woman should begin her weight-bearing exercise progressively so her bones could adapt to exercise and activity? Did they determine that this adaptation is necessary because of bone deterioration as a result of the aging process and lack of previous weight-bearing activity?

Chapter 3 Emergency Procedures

<u>After completing this chapter the student should be able to:</u>

- **Describe the signs, symptoms, and management of potentially life-threatening conditions**
- **Identify preventative measures to reduce the risk of life-threatening conditions**
- **Indicate major components of an emergency procedures plan**
- **Describe the procedures and techniques used in a primary and secondary injury assessment**
- **Identify emergency conditions that warrant immediate action by emergency medical services (EMS)**
- **Describe proper procedures to transport a seriously injured individual**

I. Key Terms

<u>Instructions:</u> *Instruct the students to define the following terms.*

Primary survey
Secondary survey
Triage
Emergency plan
Sign
Symptom
Vital signs
Unconsciousness
Partial airway obstruction
Total airway obstruction
Dyspnea
Apnea
Diastole
Systole
Cyanosis
Pallor
Rubor
Pupillary light reflex
Diplopia
Syncope
Crepitus
Decerebrate rigidity
Decorticate rigidity
Acclimatization
Hyperthermia
Hypothermia
Heat cramps
Cold urticaria
Cold diuresis
Diuretics
Raynaud's phenomenon
Hemophilia
Hemostasis
Ad libitum

II. Simulations

Instructions: *Divide the students into groups of three with one student being the injured athlete, another the athletic trainer, and the third student an observer. Have the students exchange roles from simulation to simulation as they perform the following simulated experiences.*

1 **While participating in the Senior Games, an elderly man begins to complain of chest pains after his swimming event. What questions should be asked to determine the extent of his complaint?**

1A. After questioning the senior athlete, you have determined that he may be experiencing a heart attack. How will you handle this situation?

2 **You have been called onto the field during a football game. After completing a primary and secondary survey, you suspect the player may have a lower leg fracture. Demonstrate the immediate first-aid procedures for this injury.**

2A. After calling EMS and immobilizing the lower leg, think for a minute or two about what possible complications might occur as a result of this traumatic injury. What are these complications? How can you reduce their incidence?

3 **A wrestler leaves the mat during the match because of heavy and deep breathing. He is somewhat dizzy, disoriented, and is sweating profusely. What condition may be present, and what is your immediate reaction?**

3A. The wrestler is experiencing heat exhaustion. What signs and symptoms would lead you to believe the condition is deteriorating into heat stroke? How can you lessen the risk of this occurring?

4 **A downhill skier is complaining of numbness and pain in the fingers and toes. Upon observation, you notice these areas are red and swollen, yet cold to the touch. What condition may be present? How should it be treated?**

4A. What signs and symptoms would indicate the presence of deep frostbite?

5 **A gymnast slipped off the springboard on an approach to a vault and collided full force into the vaulting horse. The individual is now lying on the floor motionless. What immediate care should be provided to this individual? How should additional help be summoned?**

5A. In initiating the facility's emergency procedures plan, what priorities need to be assessed to determine if any life-threatening condition is present?

5B. The gymnast was not moving as you approached. As you moved closer, however, the individual groans and moves an arm. You have determined that breathing and circulation are present. The gymnast is somewhat lethargic. Breathing is shallow, but pulse is normal. Proceed to the secondary survey but continue to monitor vitals signs. What are the vital signs?

5C. The gymnast reported pain on the left side of the chest and increased pain during deep inhalations. There is discoloration present on the lower left side of the anterior chest wall. Palpation elicited pain in the region of the ninth and tenth rib on the lateral side and increased with compression on the sternum. Muscle strength and sensation in the hands and feet appear normal. Should you activate EMS?

5D. What type of information should be provided to the EMS upon arrival at the scene? Should an injury report form be completed?

III. Situations

__Instructions:__ *Have each student work with a partner to cooperatively analyze and answer the following situations.*

1. You are watching a field hockey game when a player stops running and suddenly grabs the throat with both hands and appears to be choking. The athlete is becoming cyanotic. How will you handle this situation?

2. You entered the locker room to find an individual lying unconscious on the floor. Think quickly about what conditions may cause unconsciousness. What are they?

3. A second baseman collided with a runner and was cleated across the front of the shin. The area is bleeding profusely. How will you control bleeding and decrease the risk of infection? What guidelines will determine if the individual can reenter the game?

4. After a kick toward the goal, a soccer player lands in a fire ant bed. The player gets up and continues playing; however, you notice the athlete's skin becoming red and swollen. The player is having trouble breathing and feels lethargic. What do you suspect is occurring, and how will you handle this situation?

III. Situations (Cont'd)

5. You are responsible for measuring the heat stress index prior to football practice. How is this measured? What activity should be used to prevent heat illnesses? In addition to monitoring the heat stress index, what other steps can be taken to decrease the risk of heat emergencies?

6. You have been asked to speak to a group of hikers who are going backpacking in the winter. What suggestions might you provide to prevent hypothermia during the trip?

7. A football player is down on the field. Because of the mechanism of injury, you suspect a possible head or neck injury. As you arrive, you notice the player is having difficulty breathing, and you have determined it is necessary to gain access to the airway. Demonstrate how you would open the airway in this situation. What techniques or tests would you perform to determine a possible neurological injury?

IV. Special Tests

Instructions: *Have the students work with a partner to perform the following special tests and explain the rational for each test.*

-Blood pressure measurement
-Respiration rate measurement
-Response to verbal and motor commands
-Pulse rate measurement
-Pupil reaction

V. Teaching Strategies

1. Invite an emergency medical technician (EMT) to class to demonstrate the procedures used to move an injured athlete.

2. Divide the students into groups and have them practice splinting various body parts.

3. Invite an OSHA representative to class to discuss human immunodeficiency virus/ hepatitis B virus prevention and universal safety precautions in the work environment.

4. Have the students take part in a cardiopulmonar resuscitation (CPR) course and receive their CPR certification.

5. Have the students design an emergency protocol plan for a specific athletic event or practice site.

Instructor's Key

I. Key Terms

Primary survey — — — — Immediate assessment to determine unresponsiveness and status of the ABCs

Secondary survey — — — Detailed head-to-toe assessment to detect medical and injury related problems that if unrecognized and untreated could become life-threatening

Triage — — — — — — — — — — Assessing all injured individuals to determine priority of care

Emergency plan — — — — A process that activates emergency health care services of the facility and community

Sign — — — — — — — — — — — Objective measurable physical finding that you hear, feel, see, or smell during the assessment

Symptom — — — — — — — — Subjective information provided by an individual regarding their perception of the problem

Vital signs — — — — — — — Objective measurements of pulse, respirations, blood pressure, and skin temperature indicating normal body function

Unconsciousness — — — — Impairment of brain function whereby the individual lacks conscious awareness and is unable to respond to superficial sensory stimuli

Partial airway obstruction — Choking where the individual has some air exchange in the lungs and is able to cough

Total airway obstruction — Choking where the individual has no air passing through vocal cords and is unable to speak or cough

Dyspnea — — — — — — — — — Labored or difficult breathing

Apnea — — — — — — — — — — Temporary cessation of breathing

Diastole — — — — — — — — — Residual pressure in the aorta between heart beats

Systole — — — — — — — — — Pressure in the aorta when the left ventricle contracts

I. Key Terms (Con't)

Cyanosis — — — — — — — —	A dark bluish or purple tinge to the skin due to deficient oxygen in the blood
Pallor — — — — — — — — —	Skin ashen or pale in color
Rubor — — — — — — — — —	Skin reddish in color
Pupillary light reflex — —	Rapid constriction of pupils when exposed to intense light
Diplopia — — — — — — — —	Double vision
Syncope — — — — — — — —	Fainting or light-headedness
Crepitus — — — — — — — —	Cracking or grating sound heard during palpation that indicates a possible fracture
Decerebrate rigidity — — —	Extension of all four extremities
Decorticate rigidity — — —	Extension of the legs with flexion of the elbows, wrists, and fingers
Acclimatization — — — —	Physiologic adaptations of an individual to a different environment, especially climate or altitude
Hyperthermia — — — — —	Elevated body temperature
Hypothermia — — — — — —	Decreased body temperature
Heat cramps — — — — — —	Painful involuntary muscle spasms caused by excessive water and electrolyte loss
Cold urticaria — — — — —	Condition characterized by redness, itching, and large blister-like wheals on skin that is exposed to cold
Cold diuresis — — — — — —	Excretion of urine in cold weather due to blood being shunted away from the skin to the core to maintain vascular volume
Diuretics — — — — — — — —	Drugs that promote the excretion of urine
Raynaud's phenomenon —	Condition characterized by intermittent bilateral attacks of ischemia of the fingers or toes, marked by severe pallor, numbness, and pain

Hemophilia ——————— Inability of blood to clot, which can lead to excessive blood loss

Hemostasis ——————— The state of equilibrium within the body's various tissues and systems

Ad libitum ——————— At pleasure or at will

II. Simulations

1 Heart Attack Victim

Did the students' questions include:

- pain originating behind the sternum and radiating into either or both arms, neck, jaws, teeth, or upper back
- shortness of breath, nausea, and a feeling of impending doom
- past history of heart problems

1A. Did the students determine that the senior athlete may be experiencing a heart attack and summon EMS immediately?

2 Lower Leg Fracture

Did the immediate first-aid procedures for the football player's lower leg fracture include:

- checking for a distal pulse and cutaneous sensation
- immobilizing the lower leg with a splint above the knee and below the ankle
- elevating the lower leg after immobilization
- monitoring vital signs
- activating EMS or transporting to a physician

2A. Did the students determine that a complication from a fracture may be shock and therefore should be treated for shock?

3 Heat Emergencies

Refer to Field Strategy 3-5, on page 75 in the text.

Did the students suspect that the wrestler was experiencing heat exhaustion? Did the treatment plan include:

-moving the wrestler to a cool place
-removing equipment and unnecessary clothing
-administering cool fluids
-elevating the wrestler's feet above heart level
-monitoring vital signs
-activating EMS

3A. Did the students note the following signs and symptoms that would indicate the wrestler's condition was deteriorating into heat stroke?

-increased temperature
-hot and dry skin
-lack of sweating
-rapid, strong pulse
-dilated pupils
-unconsciousness

4 Frostbite

Refer to Table 3-7, on page 78 in the text.

Did the students suspect the skier had superficial frostbite? Did treatment include:

- removing the person to a warm indoor location
- carefully warm the fingers and toes rapidly by immersing them into water heated to 104 to 108° F for 30 to 45 minutes
- when area is rewarmed, gently dry and apply sterile dressing between and over the digits
-cover the affected area with towels or blankets to keep the area warm
-transport the individual to medical facility

4A. Did the students determine that the following signs might indicate the skier had deep frostbite?

-skin appears blotchy white to yellow-gray or blue-gray
-skin is hard and totally numb

(Refer to Table 3-10 on page on 87 in the text; Table 3-ll on page 89 in the text; Table 3-12 on page 96 in the text, and Field Strategy 3-7 on page 80 in the text; Field Strategy 3-9 on page 86 in the text; Field Strategy 3-l0 on page 90 in the text; and Field Strategy 3-ll on page 92 in the text.)

As the first person on the scene, did the students initiate the facility's emergency procedures plan, perform a primary survey, summon help from colleagues, and would call the local EMS?

5A. Did the students perform the following steps in the primary survey to establish the level of responsiveness, breathing, and circulation in the gymnast?

- observe the individual moving or talking..call the individual by name. If the athlete is unconscious, summon EMS.
- assume a head and neck injury is present if unconscious, and stabilize the head and neck
- check circulation by taking a pulse, and check breathing by watching the chest rise and fall. If the athlete does not have a pulse and is not breathing; summon EMS and begin CPR. If the athlete has a pulse but is not breathing, summons EMS and begin rescue breathing.
- observe posture and signs of deformities or other trauma
- observe skin color

5B. During the secondary survey, did the students include:

- history of the injury (what, where, when, how questions)
- observe and inspect for bleeding, discoloration, swelling, deformities, skin color, pupil size, and reaction
- palpate for temperature, swelling, point tenderness, crepitus, deformity, muscle spasm, cutaneous sensation, and pulse
- special tests in muscular movements and blood pressure

Did the students monitor the following vital signs?

- consciousness
- pulse and breathing rate for 30 seconds
- blood pressure
- recheck the vital signs every 3 to 5 minutes

5C. Yes, since the gymnast is having painful, limited respirations, palpable pain, and discoloration in the thoracic region, EMS should be activated to transport the gymnast to the nearest trauma center.

5D. Did the students determine that the following information should be given to the EMS?

- mechanism of injury
- characteristics and duration of the symptoms and vital signs
- any muscular weakness
- changes in sensation
- treatment completed on the individual

Did the students determine that an injury report form should be completed on the gymnast?

III. Situations

1. Choking Victim - Did the students determine that the field hockey player was giving the universal distress sign for choking? Since the player was becoming cyanotic, did the students determine that a total airway obstruction was present? The students should first ask the athlete if he or she is choking. If the athlete's response is yes, the students should perform the Heimlich maneuver.
(Refer to text pages 82 and 83 for instructions on how to perform the Heimlich maneuver.)

2. Unconsciousness - Did the students determine that the following conditions may cause unconsciousness?

- respiratory distress
- hemorrhage
- seizures or epilepsy
- heatstroke
- hypoglycemia
- drug overdose
- cerebrovascular or cardiac malfunctions
- head trauma

3. Bleeding Victim - (Refer to Field Strategy 3-1 on page 62 in the text) - Did the students control bleeding by first putting on latex gloves and then applying direct pressure with a sterile gauze pad to the shin? When bleeding has stopped, the wound should be cleansed with a saline solution and covered with a sterile dressing. Gloves and gauze pads containing blood should be placed in a biohazard bag. The baseball player should be referred to a physician if stitches are required.

III. Situations (Con't)

4. Anaphylactic Shock - (Refer to Field Strategy 3-3 on page 65 in the text) - Did the students suspect the soccer player was experiencing anaphylactic shock as a result of an allergic reaction to the fire ants? Did they:

- place ice on the area to reduce the inflammation
- activate EMS
- maintain an open airway
- monitor vital signs
- treat for shock

5. Heat Stress Index - (Refer to Table 3-2 on page 70 in the text) - Did the students use a sling psychrometer to determine the heat stress index? Were the following wet bulb temperature range guidelines used to determine the extent of football practice?

Degrees in F	Recommendations
60	No prevention necessary
61–65	Alert athletes to symptoms of heat stress and the importance of adequate hydration
66–70	Insist that adequate water be ingested
71–75	Rest periods and water breaks every 20–30 minutes; place limits on intense activity
76–79	Modify practice considerably and curtail activity for unacclimatized athletes
80	Cancel practice

Were the following factors mentioned to decrease the risk of heat emergencies to the football team?

- identify individuals at risk
- acclimate gradually to the environment
- wear lightweight, light colored, and porous clothing
- provide adequate fluid hydration and electrolyte replacement
- utilize weight charts daily

6. Hypothermia Prevention - (Refer to Field Strategy 3-6 on page 77 in the text) - Did the students suggest the following steps to prevent hypothermia?

- layer clothing
- wear clothing that includes wool, wool/synthetic blends, polypropylene, or treated polyesters such as Capilene
- wear clothing that are wind resistant such as Gortex or nylon
- wear ski-type cap, face mask, and neck warmer
- wear polypropylene gloves or woolen mittens
- wear shoes large enough to accommodate an inner layer of polypropylene socks and an outer layer of heavy wool socks
- avoid getting wet

III. Situations (Con't)

7. Football Helmet Removal - Did the students determine that the football helmet should not be removed but, rather, only the face mask should be removed? To remove the face mask the students should:

- stabilize the head and neck by placing the index fingers or thumbs in the helmet ear holes and hold tightly
- with the head and neck stabilized, use a screwdriver, wire cutters, or specialized tool to remove the plastic clips on the face mask
- remove the entire face mask and mouthguard to allow easy access to the mouth and nose

IV. Special Tests

Blood pressure measurement - Refer to Figure 3.22 on page 95 in the text
Respiration rate measurement - Refer to pages 89–90 in the text
Response to verbal and motor commands - Refer to page 94 in the text
Pulse rate measurement - Refer to page 83 in the text
Pupil reaction - Refer to page 91 in the text
Also refer to Table 3-11 on page 89in the text for information on abnormal vital signs and what they may indicate.

Chapter 4 Sports Injury Assessment

<u>After completing this chapter the student should be able to:</u>

- **Identify the two main body segments and demonstrate anatomical position**
- **Define terms relative to the direction, regions, and joint motion**
- **Describe HOPS injury assessment process**
- **Define common assessment terms**
- **Identify specific components in a history of an injury**
- **Describe what is involved in observation and inspection of an injury site**
- **Identify principles and techniques used in palpation, range of motion testing neurologic testing, and special testing**
- **Differentiate between injury recognition and diagnosis**
- **Describe the components of SOAP notes and identify information recorded in each section**

I. Key Terms

<u>Instructions</u>: *Instruct the students to define the following terms.*

Etiology
Pathology
Observation
Inspection
Syndrome
Atrophy
Hypertrophy
Ecchymosis
Effusion
Dermatome
Myotome
Nerve root
Proprioceptors
Muscle spindle

Anesthesia
Hypesthesia
Paresthesia
Paresis
Referred pain
Somatic pain
Visceral pain
Goniometer
End feel
Anatomical position
Active movement
Passive movement
Accessory movement
Static position

Closed packed position
Loose packed position
Appendicular segment
Axial segment
Antalgic gait
Indication
Contraindication
Modalities
Diagnosis
Prognosis
Sequela
Painful arc
Valgus
Varus

II. Simulations

Instructions: *Divide the students into groups of three with one student being the injured athlete, another the athletic trainer, and the third student an observer. Have the students exchange roles from simulation to simulation as they perform the following simulated experiences.*

1 **A middle-aged tennis player is complaining of a dull, aching pain on the lateral side of the elbow. It is particularly bothersome after activity has stopped. What subjective information should be gathered to help develop a history of this injury?**

lA. A history has determined that the tennis player is 52 years old and is a recreational player who plays two to three matches per week. The primary complaint is a dull, aching pain on the outside of the right elbow after completing a match. Pain is rated as a 7 on a 10-point scale and 8 when an object has to lifted. Pain persists two hours after play has ceased. This time is reduced when ice is applied to the elbow. There is no recollection of injury but pain has been present for the past three months. A physician has never been consulted about the injury. Continue assessment of the injury by performing observation and inspection procedures.

lB. During observation and inspection, the tennis player was able to perform all gross motor movements and had good posture and a normal gait. Visual inspection showed only slight redness and swelling on the lateral side of the elbow. Perform palpation.

lC. Palpation revealed warmth and slight swelling over the lateral elbow. Point tenderness was elicited directly over the lateral epicondyle of the humerus and in the soft muscle mass on the proximal forearm. All fracture tests were negative. Perform special tests.

lD. The tennis player complained of dull, aching pain on the lateral aspect of the elbow that increased after activity stopped. The painful site was isolated, and all stress tests were negative, except resisted wrist extension. This muscular movement was weak and painful. What does this positive test indicate? Does the tennis player need to see a physician?

lE. After rehabilitating the elbow of the tennis player, it is time to perform functional testing. Demonstrate functional progression for this injury.

2 **A volleyball player reports to practice with low back pain that has been bothersome for the past 2 weeks. Perform a scan examination on this individual.**

2A. The scan examination reveals limitations in trunk rotation and pain during a straight leg raise. Continue the assessment with an examination of the volleyball player's posture.

III. Situations

Instructions: *Have each student work with a partner to cooperatively analyze and answer the following situations.*

1. A soccer player fell on an outstretched arm. You suspect a fracture above the elbow and have called the school nurse who wants to know the exact location of pain. How will you present this information so that the nurse can visualize the location of the injury and can assist you in taking the appropriate action?

2. A runner comes to you complaining of anterior hip pain. You would like to observe the individual standing in an anatomical position. How would you explain anatomical position?

3. A golfer reports to the clinic with wrist pain. What questions can be asked to determine the type and intensity of pain?

4. During a 10-k road race, a runner collapses. When you arrive at the scene, the runner is conscious. Since you do not know the medical history of the runner, what questions can be asked to gather a related medical history?

5. A football player sustained a shoulder dislocation. How will you determine if the injury damaged any arteries or nerves in the area?

6. A sport participant is recovering from elbow surgery, and you need to determine elbow range of motion. Demonstrate how you would measure elbow range of motion through both subjective and objective means.

7. After performing resisted manual muscle testing following a neck injury, you have found that the player has no pain during testing but is experiencing muscle weakness. From this test, what can you conclude about the injury? Should the individual be referred to a physician for further evaluation?

8. A rugby player has sustained injury to the low back area. You are asked to determine possible central nervous system damage through the use of reflex testing. What are the various reflexes and what segmental levels are tested?

9. You work at a clinic with several employees. Why is it so important for each employee to be consistent and thorough in all injury assessments and keep accurate records? Provide an example of record keeping most often used in a sports medicine/physical therapy setting.

IV. Special Tests

Instructions: *Have the students work with a partner to perform the following special tests at the elbow and explain the rational for each test.*

-Active range of motion
-Resistive manual muscle testing
-Myotome testing
-Functional testing
-Passive range of motion
-Dermatome testing
-Reflex testing

V. Teaching Strategies

1. Invite a nurse or physical therapist to class to further discuss the use of SOAP note record keeping.

2. Divide the students into groups and have them palpate various body parts to develop the sense of touch in the assessment process.

3. Using the dermatome and myotome charts on pages 127 and 128 in the text, have the students practice the patterns with a partner.

4. Using Table 4-4 on page 125 in the text, have the students practice determining loose and close packed positions of various joints with a partner.

5. Using Field Strategy 4-3 on page 117 in the text, have the students assess each other's posture.

Instructor's Key

I. Key Terms

Etiology ———————— The science and study of the causes of disease

Pathology ——————— The cause of an injury, its development, and functional changes due to the injury process

Observation —————— Visual analysis of overall appearance, symmetry, general motor function, posture, and gait

Inspection ——————— Refers to factors seen at the actual injury site, such as redness, swelling, bruising, cuts, or scars

Syndrome ———————— An accumulation of signs and symptoms associated with a particular injury or disease

Atrophy ————————— A wasting away or deterioration of tissue

Hypertrophy —————— Increase in general bulk or size of an individual tissue, such as a muscle

Ecchymosis ——————— Bruise; discoloration of the skin due to subcutaneous bleeding

Effusion ————————— The escape of fluid from the blood vessels into the surrounding tissues or joint cavity

Dermatome ——————— Area of skin supplied by the cutaneous branches of each spinal nerve

Myotome ———————— A group of muscles primarily innervated by a single nerve root

Nerve root ——————— The portion of a nerve associated with its origin in the spinal cord, such as C_5 or L_5

Proprioceptors —————— Specialized deep sensory nerve cells in joints, ligaments, muscles, and tendons sensitive to stretch, tension, and pressure that is responsible for position and movement

Muscle spindle ———— Encapsulated receptor found in muscle tissue sensitive to stretch

I. Key Terms (Con't)

Anesthesia	Loss of sensation
Hypesthesia	Excessive tactile sensation
Paresthesia	Abnormal sensation, such as numbness, tingling, or burning
Paresis	Partial paralysis of a muscle leading to a weakened contraction
Referred pain	Pain felt in a region of the body other than where the source or actual cause of the pain is located
Somatic pain	Pain originating in the skin, ligaments, muscles, bones, or joints
Visceral pain	Pain resulting from injury or disease to an organ in the thoracic or abdominal cavity
Goniometer	Protractor used to measure joint position and available joint motion (ROM)
End feel	The sensation felt in the joint as it reaches the end of the available range of motion
Anatomical position	Standardized position with the body erect, facing forward, with the arms at the sides and palms facing forward
Active movement	Joint motion performed voluntarily by the individual through muscular contractions
Passive movement	A limb or body part is moved through the range of motion with no assistance from the individual
Accessory movement	Movements within a joint that cannot be voluntarily performed by the individual
Static position	Stationary position in which no motion occurs
Closed packed position	Most stable joint position in which the two joint surfaces fit precisely together and supporting ligaments and capsule are maximally taut
Loose packed position	Resting position where the joint is under the least amount of strain

I. Key Terms (Con't)

Appendicular segment — — Relates to the extremities of the body including the arms and legs

Axial segment — — — — — — Central part of the body including the head and trunk

Antalgic gait — — — — — — Walking with a limp

Indication — — — — — — — A condition that could benefit from a specific action

Contraindication — — — — — A condition adversely affected by a specific action

Modalities — — — — — — — Therapeutic physical agents that promote optimal healing, such as thermotherapy, cryotherapy, electrotherapy, or manual therapy

Diagnosis — — — — — — — Definitive determination of the nature of the injury or illness made only by physicians

Prognosis — — — — — — — Probable course or progress of an injury or disease

Sequela — — — — — — — — A condition that may follow as a consequence of an injury or disease

Painful Arc — — — — — — — Pain located within a limited number of degrees in the range of motion

Valgus — — — — — — — — — Denoting a deformity in which the distal body part angulates away from the middle of the body

Varus — — — — — — — — — Denoting a deformity in which the distal body part angulates toward the midline of the body

II. Simulations

1 Elbow Injury Assessment

(Refer to Field Strategies 4-1 on text page 110 and 4-2 on text page 115)

Did the students ask subjective information to determine a history of the elbow injury?

- primary complaint; current nature, location, and onset of condition
- mechanism of injury; how did the condition occur and when did it occur
- extent of pain or disability due to injury; sport and non sport participation activities
- type of pain; stabbing, aching, radiating, intermittent, how long does the pain last, what aggravates or alleviates pain
- type of symptoms; location, onset, severity, frequency, and duration
- previous injuries to the area
- related medical history
- previous treatment and use of medications

1A. Did the students observe and bilaterally inspect for the following?

- consciousness and body language
- individual's willingness to move
- scan examination
- deformity
- swelling
- discoloration
- scars that might indicate previous surgery

1B. Did the students palpate bilaterally for:

- temperature
- swelling
- point tenderness
- crepitus
- deformity
- muscle spasm
- cutaneous sensation
- pulse

1C. Did the students perform the following special tests bilaterally?

- active and passive elbow movement
- resisted manual muscle testing of the elbow musculature
- neurological testing
- stress testing for elbow ligamentous integrity
- functional testing

1 Elbow Injury Assessment (Con't)

1D. If the students recognized the tennis player's injury as a mild muscle strain of the wrist extensors, they are correct. Pain and weakness have affected normal activities of daily living, but no joint instability is present. This individual does not need to see a physician at this time but needs an appropriate treatment and rehabilitation program.

lE. Did the students have the tennis player perform the sport skills associated with tennis (forehand, serve, backhand) at low intensity and frequency progressing to higher intensity and frequency?

2 Low Back Pathology Assessment

(Refer to Field Strategy 4-3 on page 117 in the text)

Did the students' scan examination include gross motor movements of the neck, trunk, and extremities such as:
- looking up at the ceiling, looking down, and neck rotation
- forward bending and trunk rotation
- straight leg raises

2A. Did the postural examination include observation of:
- spinal curve abnormalities
- anterior, posterior, and lateral views of the body looking for proper alignment of anatomical structures
- general symmetry of the shoulders, hips, and knees

III. Situations

l. Directional Terms - (Refer to Table 4-1 on page 106 to 107 in the text) - When the students reported the location of the pain to the school nurse, did they use directional and anatomical terms such as 2 inches proximal to the elbow joint particularly on the medial aspect of the humerus?

2. Anatomical Position - Did the students instruct the individual to stand erect facing forward with the arms at the side of the body with the palms facing forward?

3. Pain Assessment - (Refer to Table 4-2 on page 114 in the text) - Did the students determine the type and degree of pain by asking the golfer the following questions?

III. Situations (Con't)

Is the pain:

- constant or intermittent
- dull or sharp
- radiating or referred
- localized or diffused
- bothersome after activity, during activity, or all the time
- does it wake them up at night

Does rest help relieve the pain? What activities increase/decrease the pain? How long does the pain last?

Using a scale of 1 to 10 with 10 being severe, when the pain begins, how severe is it and how long does it usually last?

4. Related Medical History - To obtain a related medical history on the runner, did the students ask if the runner had any previous:

- respiratory or vascular problems
- heat illness
- seizures
- chronic medical problems
- loss of consciousness or head injuries

5. Vascular and Nerve Assessment - (Refer to Figure 4-18 on page 127 in the text) - To rule out major artery involvement with the football player's shoulder injury, did the students check for a distal radial pulse?

To rule out nerve involvement, did the students test cutaneous sensation by assessing dermatome function? Did they:

- ask the individual to close both eyes
- run their fingers along both sides of the arm and shoulder and ask if it feels the same on both sides
- complete this same procedure on the uninjured shoulder and arm

6. Elbow Range of Motion - (Refer to Figure 4-15 on page 122 in the text) - To determine elbow range of motion subjectively, did the students have the athlete perform elbow flexion and extension and compare the motions bilaterally?

To determine elbow range of motion objectively, did the student use a goniometer? Did they:

- place the stationary arm parallel to the proximal bone
- coincide the axis of the goniometer with the joint axis of the elbow
- place the moving arm parallel to the distal bone

III. Situations (Con't)

7. Myotome Testing - (Refer to Table 4-6 on page 126 in the text and Table 4-7 on page 128 in the text) - Because there was no pain on resisted manual muscle testing but there was weakness, did the students determine that this could indicate nerve involvement and that the individual should be referred to a physician for further evaluation?

8. Reflex Testing - (Refer to Table 4-8 on page 129 in the text) - To determine central nervous system damage by way of reflex testing for the low back injury, did the students test the deep tendon patella reflex knee jerk? To perform the knee jerk reflex test, the students should strike the patella tendon with a reflex hammer. Deep tendon reflexes tend to be diminished or absent when the specific nerve root being tested is damaged.

9. SOAP Notes - (Refer to Table 4-9 on page 132 in the text) - Did the students determine that it is extremely important for all employees to use a uniform method of documentation to verify services rendered and to record patient evaluation, progress, and assessment, particularly when numerous individuals are involved in the patient's rehabilitation program? Did the students provide the SOAP note format for a record keeping method?

IV. Special Tests

Refer to text pages 119–130.

Chapter 5 Therapeutic Exercise and Therapeutic Modalities

After completing this chapter the student should be able to:

- **Identify the five theoretical emotional stages an individual progresses through when confronted with a disabling injury**
- **Identify and describe the process in designing a therapeutic exercise program**
- **Explain the four phases of therapeutic exercise programs, goals, and methodology of implementation**
- **List the criteria used to clear an individual to return to full participation in sport**
- **Describe the major groups of modalities, indications and contraindications for their use, and their application to manage inflammation and promote healing**
- **Describe how nutrition can enhance healing**

I. Key Terms

Instructions: *Instruct the students to define the following terms.*

Indication
Contraindication
Cryotherapy
Cryokinetics
Cold allergies
Hunting response
Thermotherapy
Hyperemia
Wheal
Current
Voltage
Cathode
Anode
Cavitation
Phonophoresis
Iontophoresis
Therapeutic drugs
Analgesic
Analgesic effect
Anesthetics
Antipyresis
Counterirritant
Salicylates
Contracture
Flexibility
Ballistic stretching
Static stretching
Active inhibition
Reciprocal inhibition
Proprioceptive neuromuscular facilitation
Hypomobility
Hypermobility
Overload principle
Agonist
Antagonist
Strength
Muscular power
Muscular endurance
Sticking point
Kinetics
Kinematic chains
Plyometric training
Coordination
Raynaud's phenomenon
Valsalva effect

II. Simulations

Instructions: *Divide the students into groups of three with one student being the injured athlete, another the athletic trainer, and the third student an observer. Have the students exchange roles from simulation to simulation as they perform the following simulated experiences.*

1 **A basketball player has sustained a season-ending knee injury. How might this individual psychologically react to this injury? What impact might the player's feelings have on his/her motivation to recover from this injury?**

1A. The basketball player is depressed and refuses to accept that the injury is season ending. What can you do to help the basketball player overcome these feelings and other emotions that might hinder his/her progress in the therapeutic exercise and rehabilitation program?

2 **A lacrosse player has sustained an acromioclavicular sprain of the shoulder and is now ready to begin therapeutic exercise. What is the first step the athletic trainer must perform to initiate the rehabilitation process? How does the trainer accomplish this using the SOAP note format?**

2A. Now that you have recorded the objective portion of the SOAP note, develop a therapeutic exercise program for the lacrosse player by performing the A portion of the SOAP note format.

2B. You have now assessed the patient and have developed both long- and short-term goals. It is now time to develop the treatment plan or the P portion of the SOAP notes. Demonstrate how you will do this.

3 **A gymnast has sustained a sprained ankle. Demonstrate Phase I of the therapeutic exercise program.**

3A. The acute inflammatory symptoms have been controlled using the PRICE principles. Demonstrate what exercises can be used to increase range of motion of the injured ankle and enhance healing.

3B. You and the gymnast are having a difficult time in achieving increased ankle range of motion. What might be causing this inhibition?

3 **(Con't)**
A gymnast has sustained a sprained ankle. Demonstrate Phase I of the therapeutic exercise program.

3C. The gymnast has regained pain-free range of motion of the injured ankle joint. Can the gymnast return to practice at this time? Why? Does the gymnast need to continue the rehabilitation process? If yes, explain and demonstrate what the gymnast will be doing in the next phase of the rehabilitation program.

3D. The gymnast has completed Phase III of the rehabilitation process and is ready to return to activity. Explain and demonstrate how the gymnast will functionally return to activity.

3E. What criteria will be used to determine if the gymnast is ready to return to full activity and competition?

3F. During the rehabilitation process, should the gymnast be concerned about nutrition and diet? Why?

4 **A runner has sustained a stress fracture of the foot. The physician suggests no weight-bearing activity for 1 week. Explain and demonstrate how to fit the runner with crutches.**

4A. After two days of being on crutches, the runner is getting aggravated and bored. What type of activity can the athlete do to maintain cardiovascular conditioning and relieve boredom?

III. Situations

<u>Instructions:</u> *Have each student work with a partner to cooperatively analyze and answer the following situations.*

1. A tennis player has sustained a mild chronic strain to the wrist extensors. What long- and short-term goals might you and the player establish for the therapeutic exercise program?

2. A wrestler has been in a therapeutic exercise program for the past month for a shoulder injury. How is progress monitored in the program? What techniques may be used to motivate the individual to work harder?

III. Situations (Con't)

3. A diver hit a foot on the board and you have applied the PRICE principle. What are the concepts behind the PRICE principle, and why is it used with an acute injury?

4. A hurdler sustained a strain to a hamstring muscle. There are no available modalities to use to decrease the muscle spasm and to assist in muscle relaxation. Without the availability of therapeutic modalities, explain and demonstrate how the athlete can relax the hamstring muscle.

5. After working on range of motion for several days, a baseball pitcher is having problems regaining active elbow flexion. Full flexion, however, can be gained through passive means. What can the pitcher do to achieve active full flexion?

6. A group of dancers has been doing ballistic stretching for years. What strategies can you use to explain that ballistic stretching is actually detrimental to flexibility and that static stretching is more optimal? Explain the guidelines used while doing static stretching?

7. The punter on the football team wants to increase flexibility of the hamstrings. Explain and demonstrate how proprioceptive neuromuscular facilitation (PNF) stretching can help accomplish this.

8. You are a high school athletic trainer with a limited budget. What type of rehabilitative equipment can you purchase to increase muscle strength, endurance, and power without overextending your budget?

9. A basketball player has sustained a quadriceps strain and is now in Phase III of the rehabilitation process. Explain and demonstrate what exercises can be used to increase muscular power?

10. A running back has undergone surgery to repair a menisci injury. The supervising physician has suggested closed chain exercises. Why? Explain and demonstrate a few closed chain exercises that could be used in a lower extremity program.

ll. A recreational sport participant has sustained a strained calf muscle. You want to increase the range of motion of the calf muscle. What type of cryotherapy technique could be used prior to stretching to facilitate the stretching program? Why are these effective?

12. A volleyball player sustained a jammed finger and is in Phase II of the therapeutic exercise program. What type of thermotherapy program can be used to supplement the program? How will you administer this modality?

III. Situations (Con't)

13. A baseball player is suffering from chronic biceps tendinitis. The physician has recommended a modality that will produce a deep thermal effect. What modality will you choose? Why? What contraindications must you be aware of prior to applying this type of treatment? Are there any medications that a physician might prescribe for this injury?

14. A shot putter has strained a triceps muscle. After applying the PRICE principle, what other modality can be combined with PRICE to decrease pain, muscle spasms, and edema? Are there any over-the-counter medications that might aid in this process?

15. A swimmer is recovering from shoulder surgery. You want to use massage to help break up soft tissue adhesions left from the surgical procedure. What massage technique will assist in achieving this goal? Why?

16. A golfer is experiencing acute low back muscle spasms. What type of treatment or medication will be best for the golfer to relieve the muscle spasms?

17. A wrestler wants a good nutritional program to use while training and competing. What guidelines can be provided to this athlete to ensure safe weight loss or weight gain?

IV. Teaching Strategies

1. **Divide the students into pairs and have them apply various modalities to each other.**

2. **Divide the students into pairs and have them perform closed and open chain exercises for both upper and lower extremity injuries.**

3. **Invite a massage therapist to class to demonstrate the various types of massage methods used in the treatment of injuries and sport performance.**

4. **Invite a modality sales representative to class to present, discuss, and demonstrate various electrical modalities available on the market.**

5. **Divide students into pairs and have each perform PNF stretching techniques on each other.**

6. **Take the class on a field trip to a fitness center and have the fitness coordinator demonstrate various types of machines used to increase cardiovascular fitness and explain the various programs that are available.**

Instructor's Key

I. Key Terms

Indication	A condition that could benefit from use of a specific modality
Contraindication	A condition adversely affected if a particular modality is used
Cryotherapy	Cold application
Cryokinetics	Use of cold treatments prior to an exercise session
Cold allergies	Hypersensitivity to cold, leading to superficial vascular reaction manifested by transient itching, erythema, hives, or whitish swellings (wheals)
Wheals	A smooth, slightly elevated area on the body that appears red or white and is accompanied by severe itching; com monly seen in allergies to mechanical or chemical irritants
Hunting response	Cyclical periods of vasoconstriction and vasodilation after ice application
Thermotherapy	Heat applications
Hyperemia	Increase of blood flow into a region once treatment has ended
Current	The actual movement of ions
Voltage	The force that causes the ions to move
Cathode	Negatively charged electrode in a direct current system
Anode	Positively charged electrode in a direct current system
Cavitation	Gas bubble formation due to nonthermal effects of ultrasound
Phonophoresis	The introduction of anti-inflammatory drugs through the skin with the use of ultrasound

I. Key Terms (Con't)

Iontophoresis ——————	Technique whereby direct current is used to drive charged molecules from certain medications into damaged tissue
Therapeutic drugs ———	Prescription or over-the-counter medications used to treat an injury or illness
Analgesic ———————	A drug or agent that reduces the response to pain and is usually accompanied by sedation without loss of consciousness
Analgesic effect ————	Condition whereby pain is not perceived, such as in a numbing or sedative effect
Anesthetics ——————	A drug or agent that leads to an inability to perceive pain and/or other sensations
Antipyresis ———————	Action whereby body temperature associated with a fever is reduced
Counterirritant ————	A substance causing irritation of superficial sensory nerves that reduces pain transmission from another underlying irritation
Salicylates ———————	Any salt or salicylic acid; used in aspirin
Contracture ——————	Adhesions occurring in an immobilized muscle leading to an shortened contractile state
Flexibility ———————	Total range of motion at a joint dependent on normal joint mechanics, mobility of soft tissue, and muscle extensibility
Ballistic stretching ———	Increasing flexibility by utilizing repetitive bouncing motions at the end of the available range of motion
Static stretching ————	Slow and deliberate muscle stretching used to increase flexibility
Active inhibition ———	Technique whereby an individual consciously relaxes a muscle prior to stretching
Reciprocal inhibition ——	Technique using an active contraction of the agonist to cause a reflex relaxation in the antagonist, allowing it to stretch; a phenomenon resulting from reciprocal innervation

I. Key Terms (Con't)

Proprioceptive neuromuscular facilitation	Exercises that stimulate proprioceptors in muscles, tendons, and joints to improve flexibility and strength
Hypomobility	Decreased motion at a joint
Hypermobility	Increased motion at a joint; joint laxity
Overload principle	Physiologic improvements occur only when an individual physically demands more of the muscle than is normally required
Agonist	A muscle that performs the desired movement; a primary mover
Antagonist	A muscle that acts in opposition to another muscle; its agonist
Strength	The ability of a muscle to produce resulting force in one maximal effort, either statically or dynamically
Muscular power	The ability of muscles to produce force in a given unit of time
Muscular endurance	The ability of muscles to exert tension over an extended period of time
Sticking point	Presence of insufficient strength to move a body segment through a particular angle
Kinetics	The study of forces that affect motion
Kinematic chains	A series of interrelated joints that constitute a complex motor unit so that motion at one joint will produce motion at the other joints in a predictable manner
Plyometric training	Exercises that employ explosive movements to develop muscular power
Coordination	The body's ability to execute smooth, accurate, and controlled movements
Raynaud's phenomenon	Intermittent bilateral attacks of ischemia in the digits, marked by severe pallor, burning, and pain brought on by cold
Valsalva effect	Holding one's breath against a closed glottis, resulting in sharp increases in blood pressure

II. Simulations

1 Psychological Needs

Did the students use Kubler-Ross's six theoretical emotional stages an individual progresses through when confronted with grief to describe how the individual might react psychologically toward the knee injury?

- denial of the injury
- isolation of self from the team
- anger with self
- bargaining
- depression
- acceptance of injury

Did the students determine that the emotions experienced by the individual might decrease the motivation to progress through treatment, rehabilitation, and full return to activity?

lA. To help the basketball player deal with depression and other emotions experienced during the injury, did the students' plan include:

- reasoning with the individual to convince him/her that the injury is real and that further participation could lead to further injury and/or disability
- if the individual becomes angry, allow him/her to have space to vent frustrations
- motivate the individual to continue being part of the team by arranging many of the treatment and rehabilitation in the same area that the team is practicing
- develop realistic short-term goals with the player
- demonstrate progress through the use of charts and graphs on a continual basis

2 Designing an Individualized Therapeutic Exercise Program

(Refer to Table 5-2 on page 141 in the text)

Did the students determine that the first step in designing a therapeutic exercise program for the injured tennis player was to do a patient assessment? Following the SOAP note format did the students' assessment include documentation of:

- mechanism of injury
- signs and symptoms
- dysfunction as compared to the noninjured body part

2 Designing an Individualized Therapeutic Exercise Program (Con't)

2A. The A portion of the SOAP note format is assessment. Did the students' assessment include:

- analyzing and interpreting information gained in the subjective and objective portions of the SOAP notes
- identification of specific deficits and assets
- recording specific problems in a section called the problem list

2B. Did the treatment plan include the four phases of rehabilitation that comprise the therapeutic exercise program?

- Phase I controlling the inflammatory response, pain, swelling, and ecchymosis and patient education
- Phase II regains any deficits in active and passive range of motion at the affected joint
- Phase III regains muscle strength, endurance, and power in the affected limb
- Phase IV prepares the individual to return to activity and includes analysis of motion, sport specific skill training, regaining coordination, and improving cardiovascular conditioning

3 Ankle Sprain

(Refer to Field Strategies 5-l on page 143 in the text; 5-4 on page 148 in the text; and 5-ll on page 164 in the text)

In Phase I did the students:

-control swelling at the ankle by applying PRICE

-choose either intermittent compression, electrical muscle stimulation, or transcutaneous electrical nerve stimulation (TENS) as modalities to help control hemorrhage, eliminate edema, and control pain

-protect and restrict activity at the ankle by immobilization through the use of an elastic wrap, tape, brace, and/or crutches

3A. To achieve an increase in range of motion did the students:

- remove the ankle brace or splint prior to beginning exercises
- have the athlete perform both active and passive range of motion exercises as tolerated in plantar flexion, dorsiflexion, inversion, and eversion
- depending on the inflammatory response, use thermotherapy (warm whirlpool), cryotherapy, and/or electrical muscle stimulation prior to range of motion exercises
- use a cryokenetic program
- apply ice after exercise session

3B. Did the students determine that the following factors could inhibit joint range of motion?

- bony block
- joint adhesions
- muscle tightness
- tight skin or inelastic scar tissue
- swelling or pain

3C. No, the gymnast cannot return to activity because of the risk of possible reinjury to the ankle. The gymnast must restrengthen the muscles surrounding the ankle joint and move into Phase III of the rehabilitation process. The gymnast may, however, practice certain skills at low intensity if the ankle is not placed at risk for reinjury.

Did Phase III include:

- the overload principle to increase muscular strength, endurance, and power
- use of the specific adaptations to imposed demands (SAID) principle
- isometric, isotonic, and isokinetic exercises
- closed chain exercises

3D. Did Phase IV (return to activity) of the gymnast's ankle rehabilitation program include:

- muscle strength assessment
- correction of biomechanical inefficiencies
- restoration of coordination, muscle strength, endurance, and power in sport specific skills
- improved cardiovascular endurance
- progressively increase in intensity and duration of activities

3E. Did the students' criteria for the gymnast to return to activity and competition include:

- normal biomechanical function of sport specific functional patterns
- muscle strength, endurance, and power in affected limb equal to that of the unaffected limb
- normal balance and coordination
- cardiovascular endurance at or greater than preinjury level
- wearing of appropriate taping or bracing if needed
- medical clearance from supervising physician

3 Ankle Sprain (Con't)

3F. Yes, the gymnast should be concerned about their diet during the rehabilitation process. An injured individual must have an adequate diet that provides the nutrients necessary to enhance wound healing (carbohydrates, fats, proteins, water, vitamins, and minerals). In addition, a diet high in carbohydrates should supply the energy necessary to train and compete on a highly competitive level.

4 Stress Fracture

(Refer to Field Strategies 5-2 on page 144 in the text and 5-9 on page 160 in the text)

Did the students use the following guidelines to fit crutches for the runner?
- have the individual stand erect in low-heeled shoes
- place the tip of the crutch slightly in front of and to the side of the involved leg
- adjust the length so that the axillary pad is 1 to 1 1/2 inches below the axilla
- adjust the hand grips so the elbow is flexed at about 30 degrees and is at the level of the greater trochanter.

4A. Did the students suggest that the runner choose one of the following cardiovascular programs to do while in the nonweight-bearing phase of their injury?
- upper body ergometer
- cycling
- rowing
- swimming

III. Situations

1. Long- and Short-Term Goals - (Refer to pages 139–140 in the text and Table 5-1 on page 140 in the text) - Did the long-term goals for the tennis player include:
- pain-free bilateral range of motion
- bilateral muscular strength, endurance, and power
- maintenance of cardiovascular endurance
- restoration of normal joint biomechanics
- increased proprioception and kinesthetic awareness
- restoration of bilateral function of activities of daily living (ADLs)
- pain-free unlimited motion in tennis skills with the use of a tennis elbow support

III. Situations (Con't)

1. Long- and Short-Term Goals (Con't) - Did the short-term goals include:
- control inflammation, pain, and swelling
- restore active range and passive range of motion as tolerated
- protect the area and decrease level of activity
- maintain wrist and shoulder strength
- maintain cardiovascular endurance with weight-bearing exercise

2. Monitoring Progress - To monitor the progress of the wrestler, did the students include the following parameters?
- daily documentation of exercise program
- documentation of edema, hemorrhaging, muscle spasms, atrophy, and infection that might impede the healing process
- periodical measurements of girth, range of motion, muscular strength, endurance, power, and cardiovascular fitness
- reevaluation of exercise program based on documentation

3. PRICE - (Refer to Field Strategy 5-l on page 143 in the text) - Did the students' rationale for applying the PRICE principle to the acutely injured diver's foot include:
- protecting and restricting activity decreases the chance of further injury and is essential if repair and healing are to progress in a timely manner
- ice leads to vasoconstriction, decreased circulation and capillary permeability, and decreased time for blood coagulation
- compression assists in decreasing hemorrhage and hematoma formation
- elevation uses gravity to reduce pooling of fluids and pressure inside the venous and lymphatic vessels to prevent fluid from filtering into the surrounding tissue spaces

4. Specific Muscle Relaxation - (Refer to Field Strategy 5-3 on page 145 in the text) - Did the students use Jacobson's relaxation exercises to help the hurdler relax the hamstring muscles? Did they:
- focus on the hamstring while initiating an isometric contraction of the hamstring for five to seven seconds
- relax the hamstring while imagining the muscle is heavy, warm, and relaxed after the contraction
- if continued muscle tension is perceived, repeat the process

5. Active Assistive Range of Motion - Did the students determine that the baseball pitcher must use active assistive range of motion exercises to achieve full elbow flexion? Did the students assist in moving the elbow through the available pain-free motion?

III. Situations (Con't)

6. Ballistic and Static Stretching - (Refer to text pages 149–150 and Field Strategy 5-5 on page 150 in the text) - Did the student's rationale include:

- ballistic stretching uses repetitive bouncing motions at the end of the available range of motion that causes muscle spindles to repetitively stretch, but since the bouncing motions are so short in duration, the Golgi tendon organs do not fire. As such, the muscles resist relaxation.
- ballistic stretching often enhances muscles to remain contracted to prevent overstretching, leading to microscopic tears in the musculotendinous unit
- in a static stretch, movement is slow and deliberate. The Golgi tendon organs are able to override impulses from the muscle spindles, leading to a safer and more effective muscle stretch

Static stretching guidelines suggest that:

- muscle is stretched to a point where a mild burn is felt
- this position is maintained statically for about 15 seconds and repeated several times

7. PNF Stretching - (Refer to Field Strategy 5-6 on page 151 in the text) - Did the students choose to use the contract-relax technique of PNF stretching that includes:

- passively stretching the hamstring muscle and then asking the individual to contract the hamstring against an isometric resistance applied by you for 3, 6, or 10 seconds followed by a relaxation period.
- alternating contractions and passive stretching repeating the process five to eight times

8. Resistance Equipment - Did the students determine that free weights, theraband, elastic, and surgical tubing can be purchased relatively inexpensively to assist in Phase III of the rehabilitation process?

9. Plyometric Training - (Refer to Field Strategy 5-7 on page 156 in the text) - Did the students choose plyometric training to increase the volleyball player's muscular endurance? Did the plyometric program include:

- progressive intensity and frequency in exercises
- exercises such as standing jumps, multiple jumps, depth jumps, bounding, and leaping
- performing exercises on grass or other resilient surfaces
- performing exercises every 3 days to allow for recovery

III. Situations (Con't)

10. Closed Chain Exercises - Reasons why closed chain exercises are recommended include:

- multiple joints can be exercised through weight-bearing and muscular co-contractions
- velocity and torque are more controlled
- shear forces are reduced
- proprioceptors are reeducated
- postural and stabilization mechanics are facilitated
- exercises can work in spiral or diagonal movement patterns

Did the students include the following closed chain exercises as example exercises for the running back?

- flat foot exercises
- Profitter exercises
- BAPS or wobble board exercises
- sand walking exercises
- balancing on toes exercises

ll. Ice Massage - Did the students choose to use ice massage on the strained calf muscle? Ice massage is useful for its analgesic effect in relieving pain that may inhibit stretching of a muscle and has been shown to decrease muscle soreness when combined with stretching.

12. Paraffin Bath - Did the students choose a paraffin bath as a thermotherapy modality for the volleyball player's finger? Did the administration of the paraffin bath include:

- cleansing and removing all jewelry from the body part
- dipping the body part into the bath several times, each time allowing the previous coat to dry
- after dipping, wrap the body part in a plastic bag or towel
- elevate for 15 to 20 minutes

13. Ultrasound Application - (Refer to Table 5-6 on page 172 in the text) - Did the students choose to use ultrasound for the baseball player's biceps tendinitis since ultrasound provides thermal effects and is used when a deep elevated tissue temperature is needed?

III. Situations (Con't)

Did contraindications for the use of ultrasound include:
- acute and postacute hemorrhage
- infection
- over areas of impaired circulation or sensation
- over epiphyseal growth plates or stress fracture sites
- over the pelvic area in a pregnant or menstruating female
- over the eyes, heart, spine, or genitals

Did the students suggest that a physician might prescribe a prescription NSAID for the baseball player such as Indocin, Feldene, or Clinoril?

14. High-Voltage Electrical Muscle Stimulation - (Refer to Table 5-7 on page 174 in the text) - Did the students choose to use high-voltage electrical muscle stimulation for the shot putter's triceps strain in conjunction with the PRICE principle? A nonsteroidal anti-inflammatory drug such as ibuprofen (Advil, Nuprin, or Motrin) may help the shot putter's condition but should not be used for a prolonged period of time.

15. Low Back Muscle Spasms - Did the students use ice and high-voltage electrical muscle stimulation to treat the golfer's low back spasms? Did they suspect the physician would prescribe a skeletal muscle relaxant such as Flexeril, Soma, or Dantrium to help relieve the muscle spasms?

16. Petrissage - (Refer to Field Strategy 5-13 on page 178 in the text) - Did the students choose to use petrissage on the swimmer's shoulder? Petrissage is used to break up adhesions within underlying tissues, loosen fibrous tissue, and increase elasticity of the skin.

17. Nutrition - Did the students suggest the wrestler adopt the food pyramid guide for a daily diet that includes:
- 6 to ll servings in the bread, cereal, rice, and pasta group
- 2 to 4 servings of fruit
- 3 to 5 servings of vegetables
- 2 to 3 servings in the milk, yogurt, and cheese group
- 2 to 3 servings of meat, poultry, fish, dry beans, eggs, and nuts
- limited use of fats, oils, and sweets

Chapter 6 Protective Equipment

After completing this chapter the student should be able to:

- **Identify the principles used to design protective equipment**
- **Explain the types of materials used in the development of padding**
- **List the organizations responsible for establishing standards for protective equipment**
- **Fit selected equipment (i.e., football helmets, mouthguards, and shoulder pads)**
- **Identify and discuss common protective equipment for the head and face, torso, and upper and lower body**

I. Key Terms

Instructions: *Instruct the students to define the following terms.*

In vivo
Prophylactic
Diffuse injury
Focal injury
Resilience
High-density material
Low-density material

II. Simulations

Instructions: *Divide the students into groups of three with one student being the injured athlete, another the athletic trainer, and the third student an observer. Have the students exchange roles from simulation to simulation as they perform the following simulated experiences.*

1 **A pitcher was struck by a hard driven baseball to the right thigh. What type of injury do you suspect and what type of force caused this injury?**

1A. What is your immediate treatment for this injury and what type of padding will you use to best protect the thigh from another single blow?

2 **You are concerned about the various oral injuries that have occurred on your school's basketball teams. What rationale can be used to convince the coach and administration to purchase mouthguards for the teams?**

2A. The administration has agreed with you to purchase mouthguards for the basketball teams. What type will you purchase? What guidelines should be used to fit the mouthguards?

III. Situations

Instructions: *Have each student work with a partner to cooperatively analyze and answer the following situations.*

1. Preseason football camp has just begun. Explain and demonstrate what guidelines should be used to properly fit a football helmet?

2. After fitting the football helmet, what guidelines should be used to fit the shoulder pads for the football player?

3. A cyclist wants to purchase a helmet and asks for advise. What advise can you provide?

4. An individual has sustained an eye injury. The physician suggests that eye protection should be worn during sport participation. What type of eye protection should be recommended?

5. A swimmer wears soft contact lenses. What concerns would exist if the swimmer insists on wearing the contact lenses during swimming?

6. A female complains of breast pain during running. After completing a history, you find no evidence of injury. She wears a size C cup. You suspect that her pain is a result of wearing a nonsupportive bra. What suggestions will you give the runner about purchasing a sport bra?

7. A recreational softball player has sustained a moderate anterior cruciate knee sprain and has moderate instability. The attending physician suggests the athlete wear a functional knee brace when the athlete returns to activity. What type of knee brace should the individual wear and why?

8. It has been decided that all soccer players on the county's recreational teams wear shinguards. What type of material should the shin guards be made of and why?

9. A baseball player has a chronic ankle sprain that requires external support. What method of support can provide a higher level of protection for this player in all four motions? In inversion and eversion? Should the baseball player be required to follow a rehabilitation program to strengthen the muscles while using the external supportive device?

10. You are working in a sports medicine clinic as a clinical athletic trainer. During a visit to the YWCA, a woman approaches you concerning how to purchase a pair of athletic shoes. She reports having high arches and enjoys playing tennis. What guidelines will you suggest for this individual?

IV. Teaching Strategies

1. Invite a podiatrist to class to discuss various foot structures, types of shoes needed for various foot structures, and how orthotics can aid in the prevention and treatment of foot injuries and abnormalities.

2. Divide the students into groups and have them fabricate various types of padding for various types of injuries.

3. Invite an equipment manager to class to demonstrate how football equipment is fitted and maintained.

4. Invite a dentist to class to discuss the various types of mouthguards used for prevention and treatment of various oral injuries.

5. Invite a sales representative to class to explain and demonstrate the various types of braces used in the prevention, treatment, and rehabilitation of sport injuries.

Instructor's Key

I. Key Terms

In vivo — — — — — — — — — Occurring within the living organism or body

Prophylactic — — — — — — To prevent or protect

Diffuse injury — — — — — — Injury over a large body area, usually due to low-velocity, high-mass forces

Focal injury — — — — — — Injury over a small concentrated area, usually due to high-velocity, low-mass forces

Resilience — — — — — — — — The ability to bounce or spring back into shape or position after being stretched, bent, or impacted

High-density material — — Materials that absorb more energy from higher impact intensity levels through deformation, thus transferring less stress to a body part

Low-density material — — Materials that absorb energy from low impact intensity levels

II. Simulations

1 High Velocity-Low Mass Force

Refer to Table 6-1 on page 184 in the text

Did the students suspect the pitcher sustained a thigh contusion? This type of injury is considered to be a focal injury. Did they determine that the force produced by the baseball was one of high velocity and low mass?

1A. Did the students treat the injury by applying the PRICE principle? Did they choose to use padding that was nonresilient and made of high-density material such as orthoplast or thermoplast? Did they layer the padding by using a soft lower density material covered by a firmer higher density material to better absorb and disperse higher intensity blows?

2 Mouthguards

(Refer to Field Strategy 6-2 on page 190 in the text)

Did the students suggest that a properly fitted mouthguard can:

- absorb energy
- disperse impact
- cushion the contact between the upper and lower teeth
- keep the upper lip away from the incisal edges of teeth which all significantly reduces dental and oral soft tissue injuries, and to a lesser extent, jaw fractures, cerebral concussion, and temporomandibular joint injuries.

2A. Did the students purchase mouthguards that are:

- durable
- resilient
- resistant to tear
- inexpensive
- easy to fabricate
- tasteless and odorless
- clearly visible to officials

Did the students use the following guidelines to fit the mouthguard?

- submerge the mouthguard in boiling water for 20 to 25 seconds or until pliable
- shake off excess water but do not rinse in cold water
- place the mouthguard directly in the mouth over the upper dental arch and center it by using the thumbs
- close the mouth but do not bring the teeth together or bite down on the mouthguard.
- instruct the athlete to place the tongue on the roof of the mouth and suck as hard as possible for 15 to 25 seconds
- remove the mouthguard and rinse in cold water to harden the material
- check the mouthguard for any significant indentations on the bottom surface to ensure it is centered correctly

III. Situations

1. Fitting of Football Helmets - (Refer to Field Strategy 6-1 on page 186 in the text) - Did the students use the following guidelines to fit the football helmet?

-hair should be cut and wet
-helmet should fit snugly around all of the player's head with cheek pads snug against the sides of the face
- helmet should set 3/4 inch above the player's eyebrows
- face mask should extend two finger widths away from the forehead
- face mask should allow for complete field of vision
- back of helmet should cover the base of the skull
- the ear holes should match up with external auditory ear canal
- chin strap should fit securely
- the helmet should not move when the face guard is pulled up and down or side to side
- the warning label must be on all helmets and clearly visible

2. Fitting of Shoulder Pads - (Refer to Field Strategy 6-3 on page 194 in the text) - Did the students use the following guidelines to fit the shoulder pads?

- determine the player's chest size by measuring the circumference of the nipple line
- place the pads on the shoulders
- the straps should be snug enough to prevent no more than a two finger width distance between the pads and body
- the entire clavicle should be covered and protected by the pads
- the acromioclavicular joint should be adequately covered and protected by the upper portion of the arch and deltoid padding
- the entire deltoid should be adequately covered and protected by the extension arch padding
- the entire scapula should be covered with the lower pad arch extending below the inferior angle of the scapula
- with the arms abducted, the neck opening should not be uncomfortable or pinch the neck

3. Bicycle Helmet - (Refer to Figure 6-2 on page 187 in the text) - Did the students advise the cyclist to purchase a plastic or fiberglass rigid shell helmet with a chin strap and energy-absorbing foam liner that fits snugly?

4. Eye Protector - Did the students suggest an eye protector that:

- is made of polycarbonate
- has a frame constructed of resilient plastic with reinforced temples, hinges, and nose piece
- has adequate cushioning to protect the eyebrows and nasal bridge
- has 3-mm thick lenses
- meet the standards of the American Society for Testing Materials

III. Situations (Con't)

5. Contact Lenses -Did the students suggest that the swimmer not swim with contact lenses but should wear goggles because of the following:

- pool water causes the contact lens to adhere to the cornea, which reduces the risk of losing the contact lens, but also increases the risk of a corneal infection
- goggles protect against organisms in the water and irritation from the chlorine

If the swimmer insists on wearing the contacts, make sure he/she uses goggles and give instructions to:

- wait 20 to 30 minutes after leaving the water to remove the contacts
- immediately disinfect the contacts once removed

6. Sport Bra - Did the students suggest the following when purchasing a sport bra?

- it should have no irritative seams or fasteners next to the skin
- it should have nonslip straps
- it should be firm and durable
- it should be a cotton/poly/lycra fabric

7. Functional Knee Brace - Did the students determine that a derotational brace be worn by the softball player? The derotational brace is designed to control tibial translation and rotational stress relative to the femur, with a rigid snug fit and extension limitations.

8. Shin guards - Did the students determine that since the force produced by a kick to the shin or a soccer ball to the shin is a high-velocity, low-mass force, the material used for the shin guards should be of high-density padding covered by a molded hard shell?

9. External Ankle Support - Did the students determine that the baseball player could benefit from an external ankle supportive device, such as a lace-up, semirigid, or air bladder model? These devices are easy to apply by the wearer, do not irritate the skin as much, provide better comfort and fit, and are more cost-effective. Yes, the use of an external supportive device should be used in combination with a full rehabilitation program to strengthen the muscles around the ankle joint.

10. Athletic Shoes - (Refer to Field Strategy 6-4 on page 209 in the text) - Did the students suggest the following when purchasing athletic shoes for the woman tennis player with high arches?

- use retailers that employ a professional shoe fitter or someone who knows about biomechanics and foot problems
- always fit shoes toward late afternoon or evening to accommodate for any increase in size from the start of the day

III. Situations (Con't)

10. Athletic Shoes (Con't)

- wear socks typically worn during sport participation
- fit shoes to the longest toe of the larger foot
- the shoe should provide one thumb's width from the longest toe to the end of the shoe box
- with both shoes on, approximate athletic skills in the shoes
- the widest part of the shoe should coincide with the widest part of the foot
- women with large or wider feet should consider purchasing boys' or men's shoes
- court shoes such as those worn for tennis need more side-to-side stability
- individuals with high arches may prefer shoes with soft midsoles, curved lasts, and low or moderate hindfoot stability
- after purchasing the shoes, walk in them for 2 to 3 days to allow them to adapt to the feet and begin using the shoes for activity for about 25 to 30% of the workout, gradually extending the length of the time the shoes are worn

Chapter 7 The Foot, Ankle and Leg

After completing this chapter the student should be able to:

- **Locate the bony and soft tissue structures of the foot, ankle, and the lower leg**
- **Analyze the function of the plantar arches and their role in supporting and distributing body weight**
- **Describe the motions of the foot and ankle and identify the muscles that produce them**
- **Explain what forces produce the loading patterns responsible for common injuries to the foot, ankle, and lower leg**
- **Identify basic principles for preventing injuries to the foot, ankle, and lower leg**
- **Recognize and manage specific injuries of the foot, ankle, and lower leg**
- **Demonstrate a thorough assessment of the foot, ankle, and lower leg**
- **Demonstrate general rehabilitation exercises for the region**

I. Anatomy Review

Materials Needed:

SKELETON ANATOMICAL FOOT/ANKLE/LOW LEG CHARTS NONPERMANENT MARKERS

Instructions: *Divide the students into pairs and have them:*
- *identify the following anatomic structures on the skeleton or anatomical charts*
- *palpate and draw the anatomic structures on their partner using the nonpermanent marker.*

Structures of the Foot

-fourteen phalanges
-distal interphalangeal joint
-proximal interphalangeal joint
-extensor hallucis longus
-flexor hallucis longus and brevis
-extensor digitorum longus
-flexor digitorum longus
-five metatarsal bones
-metatarsophalangeal joint
-head of first metatarsal
-styloid process of fifth metatarsal
-navicular
-cuboid
-three cuneiform bones
-intermetatarsal joint
-tarsometatarsal joint

Structures of the Foot (Con't)

-calcaneus
-longitudinal arch
-transverse arch
-metatarsal arch
-spring ligament or plantar calcaneonavicular ligament
-long plantar ligament
-short plantar ligament
-plantar fascia or plantar aponeurosis
-posterior tibialis
-anterior tibialis
-peroneal longus
-peroneal brevis

Structures of the Ankle

-talus
-medial malleolus
-lateral malleolus
-subtalar joint or talocalcaneal joint
-talocrural joint
-deltoid ligament
-anterior talofibular ligament
-calcaneolfibular ligament
-posterior talofibular ligament
-Achilles tendon
-retrocalcaneal bursa
-calcaneal bursa

Structures of the Lower Leg

-shaft of the tibia
-distal tibiofibular joint (syndesmosis)
-interosseus membrane
-anterior tibial artery or dorsis pedis artery
-posterior tibial artery
-tibial nerve
-anterior compartment
-lateral compartment
-superficial posterior compartment
-deep posterior compartment
-gastrocnemius
-soleus
-plantaris
-peroneal longus
-peroneal brevis
-anterior tibialis
-posterior tibialis
-head of fibula
-common peroneal nerve

II. Key Terms

Instructions: *Instruct the students to define the following terms.*

Plantar flexion
Dorsiflexion
Inversion
Eversion
Pronation
Supination
Hallux
Plantar fascia
Metatarsalgia
Pes planus
Pes cavus
Kinetics
Kinematics
Amenorrhea
Osteopenia
Oligomenorrhea
Paronychia
Hammer toes
Claw toes
Keratolytic agent
Tinea pedis
Verrucae plantaris
Stratum corneum
Neuritis
Freiberg's disease
Heel bruise
Sever's disease
Shin bruise
Syndesmosis
Tenosynovitis
Snowball crepitation
Bimalleolar fracture
Jones' fracture
Nonunion fracture
Osteochondritis dissecans
Compartment syndrome
Chronic exertional compartment syndrome

III. Kinematics of the Foot, Ankle, and Lower Leg

Instructions: *Divide the students into pairs with one student being the injured athlete and the other being the athletic trainer. Have the students perform the following:*

The injured athlete should perform the following movements. The athletic trainer should name the muscles performing the motion and provide the normal range of motion for each movement. (Refer to pages 223–232 and 259–260 in text)

-flexion of the second to fifth toes
-flexion of the first toe
-extension of the first toe
-dorsiflexion
-plantar flexion
-inversion
-eversion

After the students have determined range of motion by subjective measures, have them determine both dorsiflexion and plantar flexion using a goniometer.

IV. Simulations

Instructions: *Divide the students into groups of three with one student being the injured athlete, another the athletic trainer, and the third an observer. Have the students change roles as they perform the following simulations.*

1 **A cross-country runner reports to the training room complaining of pain along the plantar surface of the left foot. Complete a history and observation for this injury.**

1A. After completing the history, you have found the runner has been increasing his distance and has been running more frequently on street-like surfaces. He has more pain in the morning when he awakes, and then the pain diminishes. After he runs, the pain returns. His shoes are somewhat old and worn. He has some pes planus on the left foot when compared to the right foot. There is minor swelling along the longitudinal medial border but no discoloration. Continue the palpation and special testing procedures.

1B. After palpation and special testing, you find pinpoint pain near the superior medial aspect of the calcaneus and along the medial longitudinal arch. Increased pain was present on active and resistive toe flexion. Pain also increased with passive extension of the toes and dorsiflexion of the ankle. What type of condition do you suspect? What treatment do you recommend?

2 **A guard on the basketball team went down on the court holding her ankle. After being beckoned onto the court, you find the guard injured her right ankle through a plantar flexion inversion force. She had no previous injury to this ankle. Perform an on-the-court evaluation and demonstrate how to move the guard from the court to the sidelines.**

2A. The athlete is now on the sidelines. Perform a more in-depth palpation and special testing portion of the assessment.

2B. What criteria will determine if the guard can reenter the game? Demonstrate the functional testing the athlete should be able to perform prior to reentering the game. Will any type of protective strapping, bracing, or taping be used? If yes, which technique will be used and why? Demonstrate its application. What treatment do you recommend?

3 **A middle-aged tennis player was playing on a cool day when the individual felt a sudden, painful tearing sensation in the calf, leading to immediate disability. What factors may have contributed to this injury? Perform the observation and palpation procedures for this injury. During the assessment, differentiate between bone and soft tissue injury.**

3A. After performing the observation and palpation, you find the area is swollen, point tender, discolored, and the athlete is experiencing muscle spasms. Continue with special testing.

3B. After performing range of motion and other special testing procedures, you find the athlete unable to bear weight and actively plantar flex the affected foot. What injury should be suspected? What is the immediate treatment protocol?

4 **During preseason conditioning, a volleyball player developed pain along the distal medial-tibial border that is present at the start of practice and running. The pain diminishes as activity progresses only to recur after activity ends. What factors may initiate this condition? How will you determine the difference between bone and soft tissue injury? Perform observation and palpation procedures for this injury?**

4A. After performing observation and palpation, you find the athlete has noticeable foot pronation on the affected leg and pes planus. The area is point tender but not swollen, hot, or discolored. The athlete has a dorsal pedis pulse and has normal sensory function. What injury should be suspected? How should this injury be managed?

V. Situations

Instructions: *Have each student work with a partner to cooperatively analyze and address the following situations.*

1. A defensive back has throbbing pain on the plantar side of the great toe on the right foot. The pain increases significantly when the athlete pushes off the right foot to block an opponent. What might have caused this condition? What injury should be suspected? Demonstrate the treatment protocol for this injury.

2. A basketball player has an aggravating pain in the Achilles tendon region of the left lower leg. This pain has been present for the past 2 weeks. Determine the difference between tendon and bursa injury. Determine the severity of this injury. How should this injury be managed?

3. A field hockey player's foot was stepped on by an opposing player. Demonstrate how a possible fracture to the metatarsals and phalanges should be determined. Should sensation and circulation be checked? If yes, demonstrate these procedures.

4. After wrestling practice, a wrestler complains of a dry itching sensation on his feet and between his toes. Observation reveals dry vesicular lesions and cracking fissures of the skin. What factors may produce these signs and symptoms? What condition should be suspected? How should this condition be managed?

5. A soccer player was hit on the left superior lateral leg. Although the initial pain subsided, the dorsum of the foot feels somewhat numb. Determine the difference between a contusion and an acute compartment syndrome. What complications might occur from this type of injury? What should the immediate treatment be for this injury?

6. A basketball player is recovering from a mild, second-degree inversion ankle sprain. After controlling acute swelling and inflammation, what exercises should be included in the rehabilitation program?

VI. Special Tests

Instructions: *Have the students work with a partner to perform and explain the rationale for each of the following special tests.*

-Thompson test **-Anterior drawer test** **-Talar tilt**

VII. Teaching Strategies

1. **Invite a podiatrist to discuss the use of orthotics in the treatment and prevention of specific foot conditions.**

2. **Invite an expert in the fabrication of orthotics to demonstrate the types of orthotics and how foot orthotics are constructed.**

3. **Invite a certified athletic trainer to discuss and demonstrate taping and strapping techniques for ankle and foot injuries.**

4. **Invite an athletic shoe expert to discuss the differences in athletic shoe design and construction and discuss how athletic shoes can prevent injuries and enhance performance.**

5. **Take the class on a field trip to a nearby prosthetic/orthotic company to observe how these devices are made.**

6. **Have the students evaluate each other's posture.**

7. **Using a treadmill, have the students evaluate each other's dynamic gait patterns.**

Instructor's Key

I. Anatomy

Refer to Table 7-1 on page 228 in the text

II. Key Terms

Hallux	The first or great toe
Plantar fascia	Specialized band of fascia that covers the plantar surface of the foot and helps support the longitudinal arch
Metatarsalgia	A condition involving general discomfort around the metatarsal heads
Pes planus	Flat feet
Pes cavus	High arches
Pronation	Combined motions of calcaneal eversion, foot abduction, and dorsiflexion
Supination	Combined motions of calcaneal inversion, foot adduction, and plantar flexion
Kinetics	Study of the forces causing and resulting from motion
Kinematics	Study of the spatial and temporal aspects of movement
Amenorrhea	Absence or abnormal stoppage of menses
Osteopenia	Pathological condition of reduced bone mineral density
Oligomenorrhea	Menstruation involving scant blood loss
Paronychia	A fungal/bacterial infection in the folds of the skin surrounding a fingernail or toenail
Hammer toes	A flexion deformity of the distal interphalangeal (DIP) joint of the toes
Claw toes	A toe deformity characterized by hyperextension of the metatarsophalangeal (MP) joint and hyperflexion of the interphalangeal (IP) joint

II. Key Terms (Con't)

Keratolytic agent — — — An agent that promotes softening and dissolution or peeling of the horny layer of skin

Tinea pedis — — — — — — — A common fungal infection found between the toes characterized by small vesicles, itching, and scaling

Verrucae plantaris — — — Plantar warts

Stratum corneum — — — The outermost layer of the epidermis; horny layer of cells that are dead

Neuritis — — — — — — — — Inflammation or irritation of a nerve commonly found between the third and fourth metatarsal heads

Freiberg's disease — — — Avascular necrosis that occurs to the second metatarsal head in some adolescents

Heel bruise — — — — — — Contusion to the subcutaneous fat pad located over the inferior aspect of the calcaneus

Sever's disease — — — — A traction-type injury, or osteochondrosis, of the calcaneal apophysis seen in young adolescents

Shin bruise — — — — — — — A contusion of the tibia, sometimes referred to as tibial periostitis

Syndesmosis — — — — — — A joint where the opposing surfaces are joined together by fibrous connective tissue

Tenosynovitis — — — — — — Inflammation of the inner lining of the tendon sheath caused by friction between the tendon and the sheath

Snowball crepitation — — Sound similar to that heard when crunching snow into a snowball, indicating presence of tenosynovitis

Bimalleolar fracture — — Fractures of both the medial and lateral malleolus

Bipartite — — — — — — — — Having two parts

Jones fracture — — — — A transverse stress fracture of the proximal shaft of the fifth metatarsal

Nonunion fracture — — — A fracture where healing is delayed or fails to unite at all

II. Key Terms (Con't)

Osteochondritis dissecans — Inflammation of both bone and cartilage that can split the pieces into the joint, resulting in loss of blood supply to the fragments

Compartment syndrome — A condition where increased intramuscular pressure is brought on by activity that impedes blood flow and function of tissues within that compartment

Chronic exertional Compartment syndrome — Intermittent excessive pressure that reduces blood flow through a muscular compartment causing pain and possible paresthesia

III. Kinematics of the Foot, Ankle, and Lower Leg

Movement	Muscles	Normal ROM
Flexion of second to fifth toes	Flexor digitorum longus	
Flexion of first toe	Flexor hallucis longus	
Extension of first toe	Extensor hallucis longus	
Dorsiflexion	Extensor hallucis longus	20°
	Anterior tibialis	
	Extensor digitorum longus	
Plantar flexion	Gastrocnemius	30° - 50°
	Soleus	
	Plantaris	
Supination	Tibialis posterior	45° - 60°
	Tibialis anterior	
Pronation	Peroneals	15° - 30°

Refer to Table 7-1 on page 228 and pages 259 to 260 in the text.

IV. Simulations

1 Plantar fasciitis

During the history did the students:

- determine if the injury was chronic or acute
- ask questions about training regimen (time, distance, surface, progression)
- ask questions about type of shoes
- ask where, when, how the injury occurred
- ask about previous injury, treatment, or medications
- ask about the type of pain the athlete is experiencing (dull, sharp, radiating, constant, intermittent, localized, general, increased during activity)
- ask if rest helped the injury

1 Plantar fasciitis (Con't)

1A. Did the students palpate the following structures for point tenderness, swelling, deformity, sensation, or other signs of trauma?

-metatarsal arch
-transverse arch
-longitudinal arch
-calcaneous
-plantar surface of foot

During the special tests did the students:

- perform the squeeze test for possible stress fracture of metatarsals
- have the athlete flex and extend toes as well as plantar flex and dorsiflex the ankle
- stretch the plantar surface of the foot by having the athlete extend the toes while passively dorsiflexing the foot
- apply resistance to toe flexion
- have the athlete walk, run, or perform other functional activities

1B. Did the students suspect plantar fasciitis?

(Refer to Field Strategy 7-5 on text page 249 for management of fasciitis)

2 Ankle Sprain

During the court evaluation did the students:

-ask why, how, and what questions
-ask questions concerning location and severity of pain
-ask about previous injury
-observe the region around the ankle with the shoe on for swelling, discoloration, or deformity
-perform special testing for fractures with the shoe on
-ask the athlete to move the ankle with the shoe on after performing a negative stress test for fracture
-remove the athlete from the court with an assistive or nonassistive carrying mode, depending on the extent of injury

2A. After the athlete was assisted to the sidelines and the shoe and sock were removed, were the following structures palpated for swelling, deformity, and point tenderness?

-metatasals
-tarsal bones
-medial and lateral malleolus
-sinus tarsi area and anterior talofibular ligament
-calcaneofibular ligament
-posterior talofibular ligament
-deltoid ligament
-Achilles tendon
-calcaneus
-palpate bilaterally

Did the students perform the following special tests?

-range of motion (passive, active, and resistive)
-stress tests for ankle and forefoot fracture
-anterior drawer test and talar tilt
-functional activities (walking, running, jumping)

2B. In determining if the athlete could return to participation, did the students rule out:

-fracture
-ligament instability
-dislocation

Did the students determine that the athlete could return to participation if the following could be performed without a limp and with very mild discomfort?

-walk, run, jump
-functional activities

Did the students use a closed basketweave taping procedure before returning the athlete to the game? After the game, did the students apply ICE? (Refer to Field Strategy 7-4 on page 245 in the text for management of lateral ankle sprains)

3 Ruptured Achilles Tendon

Did the students determine that the following factors may have contributed to the tennis player's injury?

-lack of flexibility
-lack of warm-up before activity
-lack of strength
-age of athlete
-overloading mechanism

Did the students observe bilaterally for:

-swelling, discoloration, deformity, other signs of trauma

Did the students palpate bilaterally for:

-swelling, deformity, crepitation, point tenderness, other signs of trauma

Did the students determine that bone injuries would have point tenderness over the injury site and possible visible deformity, whereas soft tissue injuries would result in more general pain?

3A. During the special tests did the students:

-perform active, passive, and resistive range of motion (if possible)
-perform stress test for bone fracture of the lower leg
-perform the Thompson test for Achilles tendon rupture
-ask the athlete if he or she could bear weight

Did the students suspect an Achilles tendon rupture? Did they apply ICE, immobilize, and refer immediately to a physician?

4 Medial-Tibial Stress Syndrome

Did the students determine the following factors could have contributed to the volleyball player's injury?

-lack of flexibility
-lack of progression in training regimen
-changing of running and practice surface
-overuse
-lack of supportive footwear

***It is difficult to differentiate between bone and soft tissue injury of this area. Treatment of either injury is the same. If the injury does not respond to the treatment, referral to a physician is needed.**

Did the students observe bilaterally for:

-deformity, swelling, discoloration, other signs of trauma
-posture abnormalities (genu valgus and varus, ankle pronation and supination, tibial torsion, pelvic tilt, short leg syndrome, pes planus, pes cavus)
-the athlete's footwear
-the athlete's walking gait pattern

Did the students palpate the following structures bilaterally for swelling, deformity, point tenderness, temperature, and other signs of trauma?

-anterior tibialis
-medial shaft of the tibia
-interosseus membrane
-syndesmosis

Did the students palpate for sensation and circulation?

4A. Did the students suspect this injury to be medial-tibial stress syndrome? (Refer to Field Strategy 7-6 on page 251 in the text for management procedures for medial-tibial stress syndrome)

V. Situations

1. **Turf Toe** - Did the students determine this condition to be turf toe? Did they determine that lack of supportive toe counters in the athlete's shoes and playing on turf were factors that may have contributed to this injury? To manage this condition did they:

-apply ICE
-use a turf toe supportive tape procedure or strap for support
-work on range of motion and strength when applicable

2. **Achilles Tendonitis -** Did the students determine that the basketball player was experiencing Achilles tendonitis rather than retrocalcaneal bursitis by palpating the Achilles tendon and retrocalcaneal bursa for:

-point tenderness
-swelling
-deformity
-temperature
-crepitation

V. Situations (Con't)

Did the students determine the severity of this injury by looking for functional limitations and points of pain as the athlete performed:
-range of motion: active, passive, resistive
-functional activities, walking, running, jumping, and so forth
-the Thompson test for integrity of the Achilles tendon

Did the students' treatment protocol include:
-apply ICE
-apply a heel lift for support
-begin range of motion and strength exercises when applicable

3. Metatarsal Fracture - To check for stress fracture of the metarsals and phalanges, did the students perform the squeeze test, compression, or distraction test? Did the students check for sensation and circulation? **Refer to Field Strategy 7-9 on page 259 in the text to determine a possible fracture of the foot and lower leg.**

4. Tinea Pedis - Did the students determine that the condition of the wrestler could be tinea pedis? Did they determine that the following conditions could contribute to tinea pedis?
-lack of drying feet after showers
-lack of wearing shoes in showers and locker rooms
-wearing colored socks when feet are wet or in wet footwear
(Refer to Field Strategy 7-3 on page 238 in the text for management of tinea pedis [athlete's foot]

5. Acute Anterior Compartment Syndrome - To differentiate between a contusion or an acute compartment syndrome sustained by the soccer player did the students:
-palpate for swelling, deformity, temperature, and other signs of trauma
-check for pulse in the anterior tibial artery and dorsalis pedis artery
-check for sensation

Did the students determine the following complications?
-loss of sensation
-decreased functional abnormalities
-diminished pulse
-contusion to the peroneal nerve
-fracture to the fibula

In the treatment protocol, did the students use ice but not compression because external compression will hasten tissue deterioration? Did they choose not to elevate the limb because of decreased arterial pressure? Did they immediately refer the athlete to a physician?

V. Situations (Con't)

6. Ankle Rehabilitation Exercises - Did the students include the following exercises in the rehabilitation plan?

-ankle alphabet
-triceps surae stretch
-theraband or surgical tubing exercises in all ranges of ankle motion
-unilateral balance exercises
-BAPS board or other proprioception exercises
(Refer to Field Strategy 7-10 on page 265 in the text)

VII. Special Test

Refer to pages 259–264 in the text

Chapter 8 The Knee

After completing this chapter the student should be able to:

- **Locate the important bony and soft tissue structures of the knee region**
- **Describe the motions of the knee and identify the muscles that produce them**
- **Explain what forces produce the loading patterns responsible for common injuries at the knee**
- **Recognize specific injuries at the knee**
- **Describe and demonstrate an assessment of the knee and patellofemoral joint**
- **Identify protective padding and commercial products to assist in the prevention and management of knee and patella injuries**
- **Demonstrate general rehabilitation exercises for the region**

I. Anatomy Review

Materials Needed:

SKELETON | ANATOMICAL KNEE CHARTS | NONPERMANENT MARKERS

Instructions: *Divide the students into pairs and have them:*
- *identify the following anatomical structures on the skeleton or anatomical charts*
- *palpate and draw the anatomical structures on their partner using the nonpermanent marker.*

Structures of the Knee

-tibiofemoral joint
-patellofemoral joint
-tibia
-femur
-fibula
-medial and lateral tibial plateaus
-medial and lateral femoral condyles
-head of fibula
-patella
-trochlear groove
-medial meniscus
-lateral meniscus
-suprapatellar bursa
-superficial infrapatellar bursa
-deep infrapatellar bursa
-prepatella bursa
-subpopliteal bursa
-pes anserine bursa
-tibial collateral ligament
-fibular collateral ligament

Structures of the Knee (Con't)

-anterior cruciate
-posterior cruciate
-coronary ligaments
-meniscofemoral ligament
-arcuate ligament
-popliteal space
-gracilis
-sartorius
-semimembranosus
-semitendinosus
-iliotibial band
-Gerdy's tubercle
-rectus femoris
-vastus lateralis
-vastus medialis
-vastus intermedius
-biceps femoris
-popliteus
-gastrocnemius
-plantaris
-tibial nerve
-common peroneal nerve
-popliteal artery

II. Key Terms

Instructions: *Instruct the students to define the following terms.*

Intracapsular
Extrasynovial
Menisci
Bucket-handle tear
Parrot-beak tear
Collateral ligaments
Valgus laxity
Varus laxity
Cruciate ligaments
Tibiofemoral joint
Patellofemoral joint
Chondromalacia patellae
Patellofemoral stress syndrome
Patella plica
Extensor mechanism
Q-angle
Screwing home mechanism
Chondral fracture
Osteochondral fracture
Osteochondritis dissecans
Larsen-Johansson disease
Osgood-Schlatter disease
Arthralgia
Hemarthrosis
Neoplasm

III. Kinematics

Instructions: *Divide the students into pairs and have them perform the following with one student being the injured athlete and the other the athletic trainer. Have the injured athlete perform the following movements while the athletic trainer names the muscles that are performing the movements along with the normal range of motion for each movement.*

-knee flexion
-knee extension
-medial rotation of the tibia
-lateral rotation of the tibia
-patellofemoral joint motion

After the students have determined the range of motion of the knee joint through subjective means, they should measure both knee flexion and extension with a goniometer.

IV. Simulations

Instructions: *Divide the students into groups of three with one student being the injured athlete, another the athletic trainer, and the third student an observer. Have the students exchange roles from simulation to simulation as they perform the following simulated experiences.*

1 **A distance runner has pain on weight bearing and mild swelling on the anteromedial aspect of the proximal tibia just below the joint line. This injury has been irritating the runner for 2 weeks. Perform a history, observation, and palpation of this injury.**

1A. After completing the history of the injury, you learned that the runner's training mileage has significantly increased during the past 3 weeks, although intensity has remained the same. However, it now hurts the runner just to walk. Observation reveals minor swelling over the area and moderate pronation and pes planus on the affected leg. The shoes are worn but still in adequate shape for the training required. Palpation reveals point tenderness pain over the medial-tibial plateau. What condition do you suspect and how will you manage this injury?

2 **A field hockey player was hit on the anterolateral side of the proximal tibia of the left shin with an opposing player's stick. Swelling occurred rapidly, but there is no discoloration or deformity noted during the observation. Perform palpation and stress-testing procedures.**

2A. Palpation reveals point tenderness over the proximal tibia area. The player has some loss of sensation distal to the injury, but the individual has full movement capabilities and a strong dorsalis pedis pulse. What is your management plan? What signs would indicate immediate referral to a physician is necessary?

3 **A basketball player decelerated, set the left foot, then forcefully pushed off the left leg to perform a right-handed layup shot. However, the player suddenly fell to the floor, grasping the left knee. The individual reported a popping sensation and a feeling of giving way in the knee. Extreme pain is evident over the anteromedial joint line. Explain and demonstrate your on-the-court evaluation for this injury.**

3A. Within minutes, rapid joint effusion and tenderness are present over the anteromedial joint line and in the posterior aspect of the knee. When performing the Lachman test, pain increased and some instability was present. How would you remove the athlete from the court? Explain and demonstrate your off-the-court evaluation.

3 Basketball Player (Con't)

3B. After completing the off-the-court evaluation, you found a positive Lachman test and positive valgus stress test. The individual has limited flexion and extension due to joint effusion. What structures at the knee may be injured and how would you manage this injury?

4

A young hockey player is complaining of an aching pain in the right knee that begins shortly after the start of practice that just doesn't feel right. Joint effusion and point tenderness over the femoral condyles is apparent after practice, but no history of an actual injury can be recalled. Explain and demonstrate what stress-testing procedures should be used with this injury.

4A. The skater has pain in a short arc of motion during resisted knee extension and internal rotation, but not with knee extension and external rotation. You have also found momentary locking of the knee during active knee range of motion. What injury do you suspect and how would you manage this injury?

5

A female distance runner is complaining of a deep, aching pain in the knee during activity. Explain and demonstrate your history and observation for this chronic injury.

5A. The runner cannot recall any injury to her knee. She has increased her running distance from 4 miles/day to 6 miles/day in the past week and has been running on varied surfaces. Pain is also present during ascending and descending stairs. After practice, she has been applying ice to her knee and taking ibuprofen. Observation reveals no postural abnormalities other than a moderate patella alta and slight joint effusion. Explain and demonstrate your palpation and stress-testing procedures.

5B. During palpation of the patella, the athlete reported pain and tenderness when you pushed downward into the patellofemoral groove. She also reports discomfort when moving the patella medially and laterally. During passive knee extension, the patella laterally deviates from the groove. Pain increases during resisted knee extension, and crepitation occurs under the patella. She cannot perform a duck walk or squat test without pain, and has a positive Waldron's test. What condition do you suspect? What factors may have contributed to this type of injury?

V. Situations

Instructions: *Have each student work with a partner to cooperatively analyze and answer the following situations.*

1. A wrestler has a history of a chronic aching, warm, swollen knee. There is no visible patella outline. Do you think the swelling is intraarticular or extraarticular? What is your management plan?

2. A female runner is complaining of an aching sensation on the lateral side of her knee that first began in her hip a week ago. Her pain increases in intensity as milage increases, when running hills, and when going up and down stairs. She also has a feeling of tightness within her knee during knee flexion. What injury do you suspect? What predisposing factors may have contributed to this injury?

3. After performing a history, observation, and palpation on a softball player's acutely injured knee, you have ruled out collateral or cruciate ligament injury. However, you still suspect medial menisci injury. Explain and demonstrate the special tests for medial menisci injury. What constitutes a positive test? Why?

4. A female soccer player was decelerating after a drive to the goal and was cutting upfield to chase an opposing player. Her knee collapses, and she falls to the ground. Observation reveals that the athlete's patella is laterally displaced. How would you manage this injury? Other than the patella, what other structures could be injured?

5. An adolescent basketball player is complaining of bilateral distal patella tendon pain. Explain and demonstrate how you would determine the difference between patella tendinitis and Osgood-Schlatter syndrome. What are the treatment protocols for each condition?

6. After a second-degree medial collateral knee injury, an individual is ready to begin active exercise as part of a rehabilitation program. List the types of exercises you would have the individual perform in a nonweight-bearing position.

VI. Special Tests

Instructions: *Have the students work with a partner to perform the following special tests and explain the rationale for each test.*

- **Lachman**
- **Anterior drawer**
- **Posterior drawer**
- **Valgus and varus stress**
- **Gravity test**
- **McMurry's**
- **Apley compression**
- **Brush or stroke test**
- **Ballotable patella**
- **Patella compression or grind test**
- **Patella apprehension test**
- **Ober's test**
- **Nobel's compression**

VII. Teaching Strategies

1. Have the students perform a lower body postural analysis on each other.

2. Invite an orthopedist to class to demonstrate both acute and chronic knee evaluations.

3. Invite a brace expert to class to demonstrate various braces used for knee injuries during treatment and activity.

4. Invite an orthopedic surgeon to discuss current surgical techniques used to repair the structures of the knee.

5. Debate the pros and cons of partial meniscectomy versus total.

Instructor's Key

I. Anatomy

Refer to Tables 8-l on page 273 in the text and 8-2 on page 274 in the text

II. Key Terms

Intracapsular — — — — — Structures found within the articular capsule

Extrasynovial — — — — — Structures found outside of the synovial cavity

Menisci — — — — — — — — Fibrocartilage discs within the knee joint that reduce joint stress

Bucket-handle tear — — — Longitudinal meniscal tear of the central segment that can displace into the joint, leading to locking of the knee

Parrot-beak tear — — — — Horizontal meniscal tear typically in the middle segment of the lateral meniscus

Collateral ligaments — — — Major ligaments that cross the medial and lateral aspects of the knee

Valgus laxity — — — — — An opening of the medial side of the joint caused by the distal segment moving laterally

Varus laxity — — — — — — — An opening on the lateral side of a joint caused by the distal segment moving medially

Cruciate ligaments — — — Major ligaments that crisscross the knee in the anteroposterior direction

Tibiofemoral joint — — — Dual condyloid joints between the tibial and femoral condyles that function primarily as a modified hinge joint

Patellofemoral joint — — — Gliding joint between the patella and the patellar groove of the femur

Chondromalacia patella —— Degenerative condition in the articular cartilage of the patella caused by abnormal compression or shearing forces

Patellofemoral stress syndrome — — Condition whereby the lateral retinaculum is tight, or the vastus medialis oblique is weak, leading to lateral excursion and pressure on the lateral facet of the patella causing a painful condition

II. Key Terms (Con't)

Patella plica — — — — — A fold in the synovial lining that may cause medial knee pain associated with trauma

Extensor mechanism — — Complex interaction of muscles, ligaments, and tendons that stabilize and provide the motion at the patellofemoral joint

Q-angle — — — — — — — — Angle between the line of the quadriceps force and the patella tendon

Screwing home mechanism– Rotation of the tibia on the femur during extension that produces an anatomical "locking" of the knee

Chondral fracture — — — Fracture involving the articular cartilage at a joint

Osteochondral fracture — — Fracture involving the articular cartilage and underlying bone

Osteochondritis dissecans— Localized area of avascular necrosis, resulting from complete or incomplete separation of joint cartilage and subchondral bone

Larsen-Johansson disease— Inflammation or partial avulsion of the apex of the patella due to traction forces

Osgood-Schlatter disease— Inflammation or partial avulsion of the tibial apophysis due to traction forces

Arthralgia — — — — — — — Severe joint pain

Hemarthrosis — — — — — — Collection of blood within a joint or cavity

Neoplasm — — — — — — — Tumor that can be benign or malignant

III. Kinematics of the Knee

Motion	Muscles	Range of Motion
Knee flexion	Semitendinosus	0–135°
	Semimembranosus	
	Biceps femoris	
	Sartorius	
	Gracilis	
Knee extension	Rectus femoris	0–15°
	Vastus lateralis	
	Vastus medialis	
	Vastus intermedius	
Medial rotation of the tibia	Sartorius	20–30°
	Semitendinosus	
	Semimembranosus	
	Gracilis	
Lateral rotation of the tibia	Biceps femoris	30–40°
Patellofemoral joint motion	Vastus medialis	

IV. Simulations

1 Medial-Tibial Plateau Stress Fracture

During the history, did the students ask:
- what, when, and how questions
- about past injury, treatment, medications
- type of pain
- changes in training, running surface, distance, mileage
- changes in footwear
- pain during activity or inactivity
- functional abilities

During observation, did the students bilaterally observe:
- for swelling, discoloration, deformity, other signs of trauma
- pes planus, pes cavus, foot pronation, and foot supination
- genu valgus, varus, tibial torsion
- leg length discrepancies
- walking gait pattern
- shoe wear

1 Medial-Tibial Plateau Stress Fracture (Con't)

During palpation, did the students bilaterally palpate for:

- swelling, temperature, deformity, point tenderness, other signs of trauma
- possible fracture

1A. Did the students suspect the runner had a stress fracture of the medial-tibial plateau? This may be due to the repetitive overuse from the increased mileage. In addition, the point tenderness over the medial-tibial plateau should have identified a possible bony injury. Did the students include the following in the management plan?

- ice to control pain
- crutch fitting
- physician referral for a radiograph
- rest from weight-bearing activities
- gradual progression back into weight-bearing activities

2 Contusion

During palpation, did the students bilaterally palpate for:

- swelling, temperature, deformity, crepitation, and other signs of trauma
- possible fracture
- sensory function distal to the injury site
- a distal pulse

During the special tests, did the students:

- test for a possible fracture to the head of the fibula and proximal tibia
- test for motor functioning
- test for nerve functioning

2A. During the management plan, did the students:

- apply ice, compression, and elevation to the injury
- continue to monitor sensation and pulse

Did they determine that the following would indicate an immediate referral to a physician?

- signs of a possible fracture
- loss of motor functioning
- further loss of sensation
- decreased or lack of pulse

During the on-the-court evaluation, did the students:

Take a quick history by asking:

- what, when, and how questions
- previous injury

Observe bilaterally for:

- swelling, deformity, discoloration, other signs of trauma

Palpate for:

- areas of point tenderness, swelling, deformity, temperature, crepitation, and other signs of trauma
- a possible fracture

Did the students ask the athlete if he/she could flex or extend the knee?

Did they perform a Lachman test for possible anterior cruciate injury?

3A. Did the students remove the individual from the court with a two-person assistive carry?

During the off-the-court evaluation, did the students:

- repeat the history
- further observe and palpate the injury
- have the athlete flex and extend the knee, looking for limitations in range of motion and noting when pain occurred
- repeat the Lachman test
- perform valgus stress test for medial collateral ligament, menisci test, and other test that might indicate injury to associated structures

3B. Did the students suspect an injury to the anterior cruciate ligament? Did they suspect other medial structures could be damagedbecause of the mechanism of injury and their close anatomical association with the anterior cruciate? Did the management plan include:

- ice, compression, and elevation
- fitting the individual for crutches
- immobilizing the limb in an appropriate brace
- physician referral

4 Osteochondritis Dissecans

During the special tests, did the students:

- test bilaterally
- have the individual flex and extend the knee, noting pain and limitations in range of motion
- look for locking during range of motion
- perform resistive range of motion testing that included extension and external rotation as well as extension and internal rotation

4A. Because of the age of this sport participant and the findings discovered during the evaluation, did the students suspect this injury to be osteochondritis dissecans?

Did the management plan include physician referral for further evaluation and radiographs?

5 Patellofemoral Stress Syndrome

During the history, did the students ask:

- what, where, when, and how questions
- about previous injury, medications, treatment
- about type of pain
- functional abilities
- if rest helps
- about changes in training and running surface
- footwear

During observation, did the students observe bilaterally for:

- swelling, deformity, discoloration, other signs of trauma
- pes planus, pes cavus, foot pronation, foot supination
- genu varus, genu valgus, tibial torsion, patella alta
- leg length discrepancies
- gait pattern
- footwear

5A. During palpation, did the students palpate bilaterally for:

- swelling, point tenderness, deformity, crepitation, temperature, other signs of trauma
- patellofemoral joint pain

During the special tests, did the students:

- do bilateral comparison
- assess strength of vastus medialis oblique
- passively extend and flex the knee while your hand was on the patella, noting any crepitation
- resistive knee extension, noting pain
- passively extend and flex the knee, observing for laterally patellar deviation
- do the patella compression test or Waldron's test
- have the individual squat or perform a duck walk

Did the students suspect this individual has patellofemoral syndrome?

Did they determine that the following conditions may have contributed to her condition?

- changes in training and surface
- postural abnormalities
- laterally patella deviation
- strength of vastus medialis oblique

(Refer to pages 291–293 in the text)

V. Situations

1. Acute Prepatella Bursitis - Did the students determine that the wrestler could have acute prepatella bursitis and that this is an extraarticular injury? Did their management plan include:

- ice, compression, elevation
- decrease in activity
- NSAIDS
- referral to physician to rule out infectious bursitis if the skin has been broken over the injured area

(Refer to pages 282–283 in the text)

2. Iliotibial Band Syndrome - Did the students suspect the runner's condition to be iliotibial band syndrome? Did they include these factors that can predispose someone to iliotibial band syndrome?

- changes in training, surface, footwear
- excessive Q-angle
- gender
- postural abnormalities
- running on the same side of the road
- hill running or stair running

(Refer to Field Strategy 8-5 on pages 297–29 for management protocol)

V. Situations (Con't)

3. Medial Menisci Injury - Did the students perform McMurry's test and the Apley compression test to determine if the softball player had a menisci injury? During their rationale for completing the tests, did they explain how both tests were attempting to recreate the mechanism of injury in pinching the menisci between the tibia and femur? A positive test would produce pain and clicking.
(Refer to pages 289–291 in text.)

4. Dislocated Patella - In the management plan, did the students include the following?
- ice, compression, and elevation
- immobilization in the position you found the athlete in
- immediate physician referral to reduce the dislocation

Did they determine that the following structures could also be injured because of this injury?
- medial muscular attachments
- retinaculum attachments
- patellar fracture or lateral femoral condyle

5. Osgood-Schlatter Disease - In determining the difference between Osgood-Schlatter disease and patella tendinitis, did the students:
- palpate the tibial tuberosity and patella tendon for pain to determine which structure was injured.

(Refer to pages 296–297 for treatment protocols)

6. NonWeight-Bearing Exercises - Refer to page 314 in the text - Did the students have the individual perform the following nonweight-bearing exercises?
- quadriceps contractions
- straight leg raises in hip flexion, extension, abduction, and adduction
- short arc knee extensions

VI. Special Tests

Refer to pages 306–313 in the text

Chapter 9 Thigh, Hip and Pelvis Injuries

After completing this chapter the student should be able to:

- **Locate the important bony and soft tissue structures of the thigh, hip, and pelvis**
- **Describe the motions of the hip and identify muscles that produce them**
- **Explain what forces produce loading patterns responsible for common injuries of the thigh, hip, and pelvis**
- **Recognize specific injuries of the thigh, hip, and pelvis**
- **Demonstrate an assessment of the hip region**
- **Identify protective padding and commercial products to assist in the prevention and management of injuries to the thigh, hip, and pelvis**
- **Demonstrate general rehabilitation exercises for the region**

I. Anatomy Review

Materials Needed:
-SKELETON -ANATOMICAL THIGH, HIP, AND PELVIS CHARTS -NONPERMANENT MARKERS

Instructions: *Divide the students into pairs and have them:*
- *identify the following anatomic structures on the skeleton or anatomical charts.*
- *palpate and draw the anatomic structures on their partner using the nonpermanent markers.*

Structures of the Thigh, Hip, and Pelvis

-femur
-femoral neck
-acetabulum
-ilium
-ischium
-pelvis
-iliac crests
-anterior superior iliac spine (ASIS)
-posterior superior iliac spine (PSIS)
-pubis symphysis
-zona orbicularis
-iliopsoas bursa
-deep trochanteric bursa
-iliofemoral ligament
-pubofemoral ligament
-ischofemoral ligament
-rectus femoris
-iliopsoas
-sartorius
-pectineus

Structures of the Thigh, Hip, and Pelvis (Con't)

-tensor fascia latae
-gluteus maximus, medius, and minimus
-gracilis
-adductor magnus, longus, and brevis
-semitendinosus
-semimembranosus
-biceps femoris
-lateral rotators
-lumbar plexus, femoral nerve, and obturator nerve
-sacral plexus, sciatic nerve
-femoral artery

II. Key Terms

Instructions: *Instruct the students to define the following terms.*

-Lumbar plexus
-Sacral plexus
-Forward and backward pelvic tilt
-Osteitis pubis
-Myositis ossificans
-Hip pointer
-Snapping hip syndrome
-Legg-Calvé-Perthes disease
-Osteochondrosis
-Thromoboplebitis
-Phlebothrombosis
-Pulmonary embolism

III. Kinematics of the Thigh, Hip, and Pelvis

Instructions: *Have one student be the athlete and the other be the athletic trainer. Perform the following:*

-knee extension
-knee flexion
-hip extension
-hip flexion
-lateral rotation at the hip
-medial rotation at the hip
-abduction at the hip
-adduction at the hip

After the students have determined range of motion of the hip through subjective means, have them measure both hip flexion and abduction using a goniometer.

IV. Simulations

Instructions: *Divide the students into groups of three with one student being the injured athlete, another the athletic trainer, and the third an observer. Have the students change roles as they perform the following simulated experiences.*

1 **A rugby player is down on the field after receiving a severe blow to the anterior right thigh. The thigh is externally rotated and severely angulated. Swelling is present, and the athlete is in severe pain. Demonstrate immediate action for this injury.**

1A. The distal pulse is strong and regular. Skin color and temperature are normal. Have you treated the player for shock? What is the next step in the treatment of this injury?

2 **Two weeks ago a football player received a severe blow to his right anterior thigh. He still complains of discomfort, lack of flexibility, and lack of full muscular contractions. Perform palpation.**

2A. You find a hard mass over the injured area. What injury should you suspect? What treatment would you recommend? How would you prevent this injury from recurring in the future?

3 **A 47-year-old woman is complaining of pain while running. Pain is localized on the posterolateral aspect of her hip near the greater trochanter and is occasionally accompanied by a snapping sensation. Perform a history and observation.**

3A. The woman has been running more hilly surfaces lately and on the same side of a downward sloped road. She has a leg length discrepancy of one-half inch and an increased Q-angle on the affected leg. What structures could be involved? Please demonstrate special testing procedures.

3B. You find the runner has limited hamstring flexibility, lack of strength in hip abduction, and a positive Ober's test. What condition should be suspected? What treatment do you recommend?

4 **A breastroker is complaining of sharp pain in the groin area. The swimmer reports sustaining an acute injury during slide board exercises. Explain and demonstrate special testing procedures.**

4A. You find pain, stiffness, and weakness in hip adduction and flexion. Straight-ahead and side-to-side movements are extremely difficult. Increased pain occurs during passive stretching with the hip extended, abducted, and externally rotated. What injury should be suspected? If this injury was not acute and the swimmer had no pain during range of motion and special testing, but still had pain, what other anatomical structures could be involved?

V. Situations

__Instructions:__ *Have each student work with a partner to cooperatively analyze and address the following situations.*

1. During takeoff, a high jumper experiences a painful snap on the anterior side of the right iliac crest. Pain is increased during palpation of the anterior superior iliac spine, during active hip flexion, and while placing the ankle of the involved leg on the contralateral knee. What injury should be suspected? What treatment do you recommend?

2. An aerobic dancer is complaining of pain over the anterior groin that increases after weight-bearing activity but decreases with rest. The dancer does not recall a specific injury. Deep palpation in the inguinal area produces discomfort. What special testing procedures does this injury warrant? What injury should be suspected?

3. A soccer player received a direct blow to the left anterolateral thigh. Immediate pain, loss of function, and mild swelling are evident. Explain and demonstrate how swelling should be controlled.

4. A volleyball player was digging a ball and fell directly onto her anterior hip. Describe observation procedures and how you would differentiate between bone and muscular injury. Will the athlete need protective equipment to return to activity? If yes, what type will be needed?

5. A middle-distance runner is complaining of tightness and a pulling sensation just distal to the ischial tuberosity. It is uncomfortable when running on level ground, but painful and tight when running up hills. What muscle group may be injured? What special tests can be used to determine the severity of injury? What immediate treatment do you recommend? Explain and demonstrate flexibility exercises for the hamstrings.

V. Situations (Con't)

6. A softball player was struck on the medial side of the distal thigh with a line drive. Ice, compression, and elevation significantly reduced the initial swelling and discoloration. Several days later, the player is complaining of an aching, burning pain and superficial tenderness over the area. What can account for this delayed burning pain? What vascular structures may be damaged? What further treatment is necessary?

VI. Special Tests

Instructions: *Have the students work with a partner to perform the following special tests, explaining the rationale for each test.*

- **Gapping test**
- **Faber' or Patrick's test**
- **Thomas' test**
- **Lasègue's test (straight leg raising test)**
- **Leg length measurement**
- **Sign of the buttock test**
- **Ober' test**
- **Kendall' test**
- **Hamstring contracture test**

VII. Teaching Strategies

1. Have the students evaluate each other's lower body posture.

2. Have the students determine leg length discrepancy and pelvic tilt on a partner.

3. Invite a hip specialist to discuss hip injuries, surgery, and treatment.

4. Invite a physical therapist to discuss rehabilitation techniques and protocols used for thigh, hip, and pelvic injuries.

5. Invite an emergency medical technician to demonstrate how best to immobilize those who suffer fractures and dislocations of the thigh, hip, and pelvic region.

Instructor's Key

I. Anatomy

Refer to Table 9-1 on page 324 in the text

II. Key Terms

Anterior pelvic tilt — — — Anterior sagittal plane tilt of the ASIS with respect to the pubic symphysis

Posterior pelvic tilt — — — Posterior sagittal plane tilt of the ASIS with respect to the pubic symphysis

Lumbar plexus — — — — — — Interconnected roots of the first four lumbar spinal nerves

Sacral plexus — — — — — — Interconnected roots of the L_4-S_4 spinal nerves

Hip pointer — — — — — — — Contusion caused by direct compression to an unprotected iliac crest that crushes soft tissue and sometimes the bone itself

Myositis ossificans — — — Ectopic ossification resulting in bone disposition within muscle tissue

Snapping hip syndrome —— A snapping sensation either heard or felt during motion of the hip

Osteitis pubis — — — — — — Stress fracture of the pubic symphysis caused by repeated overload of the adductor muscles or repetitive stress activities

Osteochondrosis — — — — — Any condition characterized by degeneration or aseptic necrosis of the articular cartilage due to limited blood supply

Legg-Calvé-Perthes disease- Avascular necrosis of the proximal femoral epiphysis seen especially in young males ages 3 to 8

Hypervolemic shock — — Shock caused by excessive loss of whole blood or plasma

Thrombophlebitis — — — Acute inflammation of a vein

Phlebothrombosis — — — Thrombosis, or clotting, in a vein without overt inflammatory signs or symptoms

Pulmonary embolism — — Occurs when a blood clot travels through the circulatory system to lodge in a blood vessel of the lungs

III. Kinematics of the Thigh, Hip, and Pelvis

Movement	Muscles	Normal ROM
Knee extension	Rectus femoris	0–15°
Knee flexion	Semitendinosus	0–125°
	Semimembranosus	
	Biceps femoris	
Hip extension	Gluteus maximus	10–15°
	Semitendinosus	
	Semimembranosus	
	Biceps femoris	
Hip flexion	Rectus femoris	110–120°
	Pectineus	
	Iliopsoas	
Lateral hip rotation	Sartorius	40–60°
	Gluteus maximus	
Medial hip rotation	Tensor fascia latae	30–40°
	Gluteus minimus	
Hip abduction	Gluteus medius	30–50°
	Sartorius	
Hip adduction	Gracilis	30°
	Adductor magnus	
	Adductor longus	
	Adductor brevis	

Refer to Table 9-1 on page 324 in the text; Table 9-2 on page 328 in the text; and to page 347 in the text.

IV. Simulations

1 Fractured Femur

(Refer to Table 9-4 on page 343 in the text)

Did the students check the neurovascular function of the leg by checking for:

- a distal pulse
- skin color and other signs of shock
- for sensory changes through lower extremity dermatome function

1 Fractured Femur (Con't)

1A. Did the students initiate the emergency medical plan by calling EMS, keep the player comfortable and in a stable position, and treat for shock? If bleeding is present, did they cover the area with a dry sterile dressing? Did they take vital signs and monitor the player's condition until the ambulance arrived?

2 Myositis Ossificans

Did the students palpate bilaterally for:

- point tenderness, swelling, muscle spasms, and deformity
- hardness or a firm mass
- an increase in skin temperature

2A. Did the students suspect myositis ossificans? Did management plan include:

- ICE
- crutches
- rest
- referral to a physician for follow-up treatment, radiographs, and prescribed NSAIDS

To prevent this condition from recurring, did the students determine that the football player should:

- not return to activity before the contusion is healed
- wear protective padding

3 Snapping Hip Syndrome

Did the students include questions about:

- present medications and treatment
- past injuries and treatment
- type of pain
- conditioning program
- type of surface
- type of shoes
- type of activities that increase and decrease pain

(Refer to Field Strategy 9-3 on page 345 in the text)

3 Snapping Hip Syndrome

Did the students observe bilaterally for:

- deformity, swelling, discoloration, muscle spasms, or other signs of trauma
- shoe wear
- lower extremity posture including pes cavus and planus, genu valgus and varus, tibial torsion, leg length discrepancy, and foot pronation or supination
- Q-angle
- walking and running gait pattern

(Refer to Field Strategy 9-4 on page 346 in the text)

3A. Did the students determine that the greater trochanteric bursa and iliotibial band could be involved in this injury?

Did the special tests include:

- active, passive, and resistive range of motion of the hip and knee
- hamstring flexibility
- Ober's test

3B. Did the students suspect snapping hip syndrome? Did the management plan include ice, modification of activity, NSAIDS, and flexibility exercises?

4 Groin Strain

(Refer to Table 9-3 on page 336 in the text)

Did the special tests include:

- passive, active, and resistive range of motion at the hip
- weight-bearing activity (running and side sliding)

4A. Did the students suspect a groin strain? If the swimmer had not reported an acute injury, did the students suspect injury to the following structures?

- bowel
- bladder
- testicle
- kidney
- abdomen

V. Situations

1. Avulsion Fracture of the Anterior Superior Iliac Spine - (Refer to Table 9-4 on page 343 in the text) - Did the students suspect an avulsion fracture of the anterior superior iliac spine? Did the immediate treatment plan include ice, rest, and use of crutches?

2. Stress Fracture of the Pubis, Femoral Neck, or Proximal Third of Femur - (Refer to Table 9-4 on page 343 in the text) - During special testing, did the students note increased pain on hip rotation and an inability to stand on the involved leg? Did the students suspect a stress fracture to either the pubis, femoral neck, or proximal third of the femur?

3. Anterior Thigh Contusion - To control swelling, reduce intramuscular bleeding and spasm, did the students apply ice with the thigh in 120 degrees of flexion?

4. Hip Pointer - Did the students observe bilaterally for swelling, deformity, discoloration, or loss of function? To determine between muscle and bone injury, did the students:

- palpate the iliac crest and surrounding musculature
- perform passive, active, and resistive range of motion exercises
- perform weight-bearing exercises

Did the students suspect a contusion of the iliac crest or a hip pointer?
Did the students apply a donut type of padding to prevent further aggravation?

5. Hamstring Strain - (Refer to Table 9-3 on page 336 in the text) - Did the students determine that the hamstring muscle group may be involved because of its attachment to the ischial tuberosity? Did special testing include:

- passive, active, and resistive range of motion
- functional testing (walking, jumping, running)

Did the students determine that the more resistance the individual could handle during resistive stress testing the more mild the injury? Did the management plan include ice, compression, elevation, and mild stretching? Did they demonstrate static stretching exercises for the hamstrings?

6. Vascular Disorder - Did the students determine that the softball player could be experiencing a vascular disorder to the arteries and veins that course through the injured area, particularly the femoral artery and vein? Did further treatment include an immediate referral to a physician?

VI. Special Testing

Refer to pages 346–356 in the text

Chapter 10 Shoulder Injuries

After completing this chapter the student should be able to:

- **Locate important bony and soft tissue structures of the shoulder**
- **Describe the major motions at the shoulder and identify muscles that produce them**
- **Explain the forces that produce the loading patterns responsible for common injuries in the shoulder**
- **Recognize and describe specific injuries in the shoulder region**
- **Describe management protocol for specific injuries in the shoulder region**
- **Demonstrate a thorough assessment of the shoulder**
- **Demonstrate proper fitting of football shoulder pads**
- **Identify protective equipment or pads used to protect the shoulder region from injury**
- **Demonstrate general rehabilitation exercises for the shoulder complex**

I. Anatomy Review

Materials Needed:
-Skeleton -Anatomical shoulder charts -Nonpermanent markers

Instructions: *Divide the students into pairs and have them:*
- *identify the following anatomical structures on the skeleton or anatomical charts.*
- *palpate and draw the anatomical structures on their partner using the nonpermanent marker.*

Structures of the Shoulder

-humerus
-scapula
-clavicle
-sternum
-sternoclavicular joint
-acromioclavicular joint
-coracoclavicular joint
-glenohumeral joint
-scapulothoracic joint
-glenoid fossa
-glenoid labrum
-subcoracoid bursa

Structures of the Shoulder (Con't)

-subscapularis bursa
-subacromial bursa
-anterior deltoid
-middle deltoid
-posterior deltoid
-pectoralis major
-subscapularis
-supraspinatus
-infraspinatus
-teres minor
-teres major
-latissimus dorsi
-coracobrachialis
-long head biceps brachii
-short head biceps brachii
-triceps brachii
-axillary nerve
-musculocutaneous nerve
-dorsal scapular nerve
-subscapular nerve
-suprascapular nerve
-pectoral nerve
-subclavian artery
-axillary artery

II. Key Terms

Instructions: *Instruct the students to define the following terms.*

-Brachial plexus
-Glenoid labrum
-Rotator cuff
-Little league shoulder
-Bankart lesion
-Dead arm syndrome
-Impingement syndrome
-Thoracic outlet syndrome
-Scapulohumeral rhythm

III. Kinematics of the Shoulder

Instructions: *Divide the students into pairs. Perform the following with one student as the athlete and the other as the athletic trainer.*

The athlete should perform the following movements. The athletic trainer should name the muscles that are performing the motion and provide normal range of motion for each movement.

-flexion of the arm
-extension of the arm
-abduction
-adduction
-horizontal abduction or horizontal extension
-horizontal adduction or horizontal flexion
-internal or medial rotation
-external or lateral rotation
-scapulohumeral rhythm

After range of motion has been subjectively measured, have the students use a goniometer to measure both shoulder flexion and abduction.

IV. Simulations

Instructions: *Divide the students into groups of three with one student the injured athlete, another the athletic trainer, and the third an observer. Have the students exchange roles from simulation to simulation.*

1 **A young gymnast lost her balance on a dismount and fell onto the point of the right shoulder. Observation reveals the shoulder sagging downward and forward. There is a visible lump in the midclavicular region. Perform palpation and special testing.**

1A. Palpation reveals muscle spasms, pain over the midclavicular area, and a positive piano key sign. Explain and demonstrate the immediate treatment protocol for this injury.

2 **A basketball player received a blow to his left superior shoulder. The player is complaining of pain over the acromioclavicular joint. Perform observation and palpation.**

2A. Observation reveals an overriding clavicle on the acromion of the affected shoulder. There is minor swelling over the joint line but no discoloration. Palpation reveals a mobile clavicle as you press down on it and it pops back up. There are no other signs of trauma. What injury should be suspected? Explain and demonstrate the immediate treatment protocol for this injury.

3 **A swimmer reports to the training room complaining of anterior shoulder pain. Perform a history.**

3A. You determine that this is a chronic injury. The swimmer reports feeling a subluxation during the power phase of both the crawl and butterfly stroke. Continue the evaluation.

3B. Palpation reveals tenderness along the anterior and the posterior glenohumeral joint. During active shoulder abduction and external rotation, a clicking feeling and discomfort are felt. During anterior and posterior stress to the glenohumeral joint, you find considerable laxity as compared to the uninjured shoulder. What anatomical structures could be involved? What injury should you suspect?

4 **A baseball pitcher reports to you with chronic pain over his right anterior shoulder. Perform observation.**

4A. Observation reveals minor swelling, no discoloration, or deformity. However, you do find the right shoulder to be slightly lower than the left when viewed from the posterior. During palpation, point tenderness is elicited over the head of the humerus. Perform range of motion and special testing for this injury.

V. Situations

__Instructions:__ *Have each student work with a partner to cooperatively analyze and address the following situations.*

1. A little league pitcher is complaining of shoulder pain. He does not recall having an acute injury; however, he is now bothered with pain and discomfort during his pitching activity. Palpation elicits pain in the axilla region. There is minor discomfort with anterior shoulder palpation. What injury should be suspected? Why? What treatment do you recommend?

2. A baseball player is complaining that his right shoulder feels "dead" in the cocking phase of the throwing motion. Pain increases during acceleration. Muscular endurance and strength are not at the level earlier in the season. Palpation during abduction and external rotation reveals a clicking sensation. What structures may be involved in this injury? What treatment do you recommend?

3. A quarterback received a blow to his throwing arm after releasing the ball during a pass. The shoulder was forced into excessive abduction, external rotation, and extension. During palpation, you find the head of the humerus to be sitting anterior of the glenoid fossa. What injury should be suspected? Would you further palpate for neurological functioning? If yes, demonstrate this procedure. What treatment do you recommend?

4. A volleyball player reports severe pain during overhand hitting drills that is getting progressively worse. The individual is unable to actively abduct the arm between 70 and 120 degrees without pain. What structures do you suspect to be involved? Explain and demonstrate special tests. How would you differentiate between bursitis and tendinitis?

V. Situations (Con't)

5. A freestyle sprint swimmer reports anterior shoulder pain that increases concomitantly with more intense workouts. There is a clicking feeling when moving through the pull phase of the freestyle stroke. During observation and palpation, you find diffuse swelling and point tenderness under the acromion and along the insertion of the supraspinatus. Movement is restricted during shoulder abduction. Explain and demonstrate special testing for this injury. What treatment do you recommend?

6. A tennis player complains of pain in his anterior upper arm. The athlete does not recall an injury. Pain and point tenderness are felt over the bicipital groove during internal and external rotation of the shoulder. How would you passively stretch the structure that passes through the bicipital groove? What injury should be suspected? What treatment do you recommend?

VI. Special Tests

<u>Instructions:</u> *Have the students work with a partner to explain and demonstrate the rationale for the following shoulder tests:*

- **Wall push-up**
- **Acromioclavicular distraction and compression test**
- **Apprehension test**
- **Drop arm test**
- **Centinela supraspinatus muscle test**
- **Anterior impingement test**
- **Transverse ligament test**
- **Yergason's test**
- **Speed's test**
- **Thoracic outlet compression syndrome test**

VII. Teaching Strategies

1. **Have the students evaluate each other's upper body posture.**

2. **Invite a neurologist to further explain athletic injuries associated with nerves of the shoulder region.**

3. **Invite an orthopedist to demonstrate an acute and chronic shoulder evaluation.**

4. **Invite a biomechanist to explain the biomechanics associated with the overhand mechanism.**

5. **Demonstrate to the class how best to evaluate a shoulder injury when a football player has shoulder pads on and is down on the field.**

6. **Invite an orthopedist to class to discuss current surgical techniques and their implications to rehabilitation.**

Instructor's Key

I. Anatomy Review

Refer to Table 10-1 on page 368 in the text.

II. Key Terms

Brachial plexus	A complex web of spinal nerves (C_5-T_1) that innervate the upper extremity
Glenoid labrum	Soft tissue lip around the periphery of the glenoid fossa that adds stability to the glenohumeral joint
Rotator cuff	The SITS muscles (supraspinatus, infraspinatus, teres minor, and subscapularis) hold the head of the humerus in the glenoid fossa and produce humeral rotation
Little league shoulder	Fracture of the proximal humeral growth plate in adolescents caused by repetitive rotational stresses during the act of pitching
Bankart lesion	Avulsion or damage to the anterior lip of the glenoid as the humerus slides forward in an anterior dislocation
Dead arm syndrome	Common sensation felt with a recurrent anterior shoulder dislocation
Impingement syndrome	Chronic condition caused by repetitive overhead activity that damages the glenoid labrum, long head of the biceps brachii, and subacromial bursa
Thoracic outlet syndrome	Condition whereby nerves and/or vessels become compressed in the root of the neck or axilla, leading to numbness in the arm
Scapulohumeral rhythm	Coordinated rotational movement of the scapula that accompanies abduction and adduction of the humerus

III. Kinematics

Refer to Table 10-1 on page 368 in the text; Table 10-2 on page 374 in the text; and page 402 in text.

Movement	Muscles	Normal ROM
Flexion of the arm	Anterior deltoid	160–180°
	Pectoralis major	
Extension of the arm	Posterior deltoid	50–60°
	Latissimus dorsi	
Abduction	Middle deltoid	170–180°
	Supraspinatus	
Adduction	Biceps brachii	50–70°
	Triceps brachii	
	Latissimus dorsi	
Horizontal abduction/extension	Posterior deltoid	130°
	Infraspinatus	
	Middle deltoid	
Horizontal adduction/flexion	Anterior deltoid	130°
	Pectoralis major	
Internal/medial rotation	Teres major	60–100°
	Subscapularis	
External/lateral rotation	Teres minor	80–90°
	Infraspinatus	
Scapulohumeral rhythm	Triceps	
	Rhomboids	
	Serratus anterior	
	Levator scapula	

IV. Simulations

1 Fractured Clavicle

During palpation, did the students palpate the following structures for point tenderness, swelling, deformity, crepitation, muscle spasms, sensation, and other signs of trauma?

- deltoid
- acromion process
- scapula
- trapezius
- clavicle
- pectoralis muscles
- sternum
- coracoid process

1 Fractured Clavicle (Con't)

Did the students do bilateral comparisons?

During special testing, did the students:

- perform range of motion exercises
- push down on the clavicle to determine stability

1A. Did the students determine that the gymnast may have a fractured clavicle? Immediate treatment should include immobilization through the use of a sling and swathe, ice, and physician referral.

2 Acromioclavicular Sprain

Refer to Field Strategy 10-4 on page 382 in the text

During observation, did the students bilaterally observe for swelling, deformity, discoloration, and other signs of trauma.

During palpation, did the students palpate the following structures for point tenderness, swelling, deformity, crepitation, muscles spasms, and other signs of trauma?

- deltoid
- scapula
- clavicle
- acromion process
- coracoid process
- sternum
- pectoralis muscles
- trapezius
- joint line

2A. Did the students determine that the basketball player could have an injury to the acromioclavicular ligament? Immediate treatment should include ice, compression, and elevation. During the history, did students determine if the injury was chronic or acute?

3 Recurrent Glenohumeral Dislocation/Subluxation

Refer to Field Strategy 10-8 on page 400 in the text and to page 385 in the text.

Did the students ask:

- where, when, and how questions
- about training regimen (time, distance, progression)
- about type of swimming stroke
- about pain (type, frequency, duration, radiating, referred, intensity)
- about previous injuries and treatment rendered
- if the athlete is taking any medications

3A. During palpation, did the students palpate the following structures for point tenderness, swelling, deformity, crepitation, sensation, and other signs of trauma bilaterally?

- clavicle
- scapula
- humerus
- acromion process
- coracoid process
- subacromial space
- glenohumeral joint
- deltoid
- rotator cuff muscles
- pectoralis muscles
- trapezius
- sensory at axillary nerve

During the special tests, did the students perform the following bilaterally?

- passive, active, and resistive range of motion testing
- anterior and posterior stress testing to the glenohumeral joint
- apprehension test

Did the students notice any limits in range of motion, pain, or weakness?

3B. Since the injury was chronic, it could be a recurrent dislocation or subluxation of the glenohumeral joint. Did they determine that the humerus, glenoid fossa, glenoid labrum, rotator cuff muscles, and anterior glenohumeral ligaments could be involved?

Did the students observe the following structures for swelling, deformity, discoloration, and other signs of trauma bilaterally? Was an upper body posture completed?

- clavicle
- scapula
- humerus
- acromion process
- acromioclavicular joint
- anterior and posterior soft tissue structures

4A. During the special tests, did the students perform the following bilaterally?

- passive, active, and resistive range of motion
- drop arm test
- centinela supraspinatus muscle test

Did the students notice any limitation in range of motion, pain, or weakness?

V. Situations

l. Little League Shoulder Injury - Because of no previous injury, pain upon throwing, pain upon palpation of the axillary region, and age of the athlete, did the students determine that this injury could be Little league shoulder? Did the treatment protocol include immediate physician referral?

2. Recurrent Glenohumeral Subluxation or Glenoid Labrum Tear - Did the students determine that the following anatomical structures could be injured?

- glenohumeral joint
- glenoid fossa
- glenoid labrum
- rotator cuff muscles
- anterior glenohumeral ligaments

Did the management of this injury include:

- ice
- physician referral
- stretching and strengthening program

3. Glenohumeral Dislocation - Did the students determine that the quarterback may have a glenohumeral dislocation? As a result, they should check for a radial pulse and neurological function of the axillary nerve by checking sensation over the middle deltoid. Did the management plan include immobilization of the shoulder and arm, application of ice, and immediate referral to a physician?

V. Situations (Con't)

4. Impingement Syndrome - Refer to pages 389 to 391 in the text - Did the students determine that the following structures could be involved with this injury?
- rotator cuff muscles
- subacromial bursa
- subacromial space tissue
- biceps tendon

Did the students perform the following special tests?
- passive, active, and resistive range of motion
- painful arc movement
- anterior impingement test

During range of motion, did the students notice limits in movement, pain, and weakness?

5. Supraspinatus Strain - Refer to pages 388 to 389 and 408 to 411 - Did the students perform the following special tests?
- passive, active, and resistive range of motion
- drop arm test
- centinela supraspinatus muscle test

Did the students suspect an injury to the supraspinatus? Did the treatment protocol include ice, rest, NSAIDS, modification of activity, and stretching and strengthening exercises?

6. Biceps Tendonitis - Refer to page 393 in the text - Did the students passively stretch the biceps tendon by extending the shoulder with the elbow extended? This injury could be biceps tendonitis, and the treatment protocol should include ice, rest, NSAIDS, modification of activity, and stretching and strengthening exercises.

VI. Special Tests

Refer to pages 402–414 in text

Chapter 11 Upper Arm, Elbow and Forearm Injuries

After completing this chapter the student should be able to:

- **Locate the important bony and soft tissue structures in the upper arm, elbow, and forearm**
- **Describe the motions at the elbow and identify muscles that produce them**
- **Explain what forces produce loading patterns responsible for common injuries in the upper arm, elbow, and forearm**
- **Recognize and manage common injuries in the upper arm, elbow, and forearm.**
- **Demonstrate a thorough assessment of the elbow region**
- **Demonstrate common conditioning exercises for the elbow**

I. Anatomy Review

Materials Needed:

SKELETON — ANATOMICAL SHOULDER CHARTS — NONPERMANENT MARKERS

Instructions: *Divide the students into pairs and have them:*
- *identify the following anatomical structures on the skeleton or anatomical charts.*
- *palpate and draw the anatomical structures on their partner using the nonpermanent marker.*

Anatomical Structures

-humerus	-biceps brachii
-ulna	-brachioradialis
-radius	-brachialis
-olecranon	-pronator teres
-medial epicondyle	-pronator quadratus
-lateral epicondyle	-triceps brachii
-capitellum	-anconeus
-olecranon fossa	-supinator
-radial head	-olecranon bursa
-sulcus groove	-musculocutaneous nerve
-humeroulnar joint	-median nerve
-humeroradial joint	-ulnar nerve
-proximal radioulnar joint	-radial nerve

Anatomical Structures (Con't)

-brachial artery
-ulnar artery
-radial artery

II. Key Terms

Instructions: *Instruct the students to define the following terms.*

Epicondylitis
Carrying angle
Volkmann's contracture
Monteggia's fracture
Galeazzi's fracture
Colles' fracture
Smith's fracture
Nightstick fracture
Ectopic bone
Tackler's exostosis
Periostitis
Fibrositis
Malaise
Little leaguer's elbow
Pronator syndrome
Wrist drop
Forearm splints
Cubital valgus
Cubital varus
Resting position

III. Kinematics of the Upper Arm, Elbow, and Forearm

Instructions: *Divide the students into pairs and have them perform the following with one student being the athlete and the other being the athletic trainer.*

Have the athlete perform the following movements while the athletic trainer names the muscles that are performing the movements along with the normal range of motion for each movement. **(Refer to pages 421–424 and 444 in text)**

- elbow flexion
- elbow extension
- forearm supination
- forearm pronation

After the students have determined the range of motion of the elbow and forearm through subjective means, they should measure flexion of the elbow with the use of the goniometer.

IV. Simulations

Instructions: *Divide the students into groups of three with one student being the injured athlete, another being the athletic trainer, and the third student an observer. Have the students exchange roles from simulation to simulation as they perform the following simulated experiences.*

1 **A tennis player is complaining of pain on the lateral side of the elbow that is exacerbated during the execution of ground strokes. Perform palpations by stating what anatomical structures could possibly be involved with this injury.**

1A. After palpating the lateral epicondyle and associated surrounding tissue and musculature, you found point tenderness over the proximal attachment of the wrist extensors, mild swelling, but no deformity. Continue with range of motion and special tests. How you will treat this injury?

2 **A football player is complaining of pain on impact with his right forearm during blocking. History reveals an acute injury. Perform the observation and palpation procedures.**

2A. After observing and palpating the area, you found no deformity or discoloration. There is, however, marked swelling and a hardend mass of soft tissue over the distal anterior arm. What injury might you suspect, and how would you treat this injury?

3 **A little league baseball player is complaining of pain on the medial elbow during pitching. Complete a history for this specific injury.**

3A. You discovered that pain intensifies during the acceleration phase of throwing, although the throwing technique appears normal. Observation reveals minor swelling over the medial epicondyle. Please continue the evaluation with bilateral palpation and special tests. What nerve might be associated with this injury? What elbow injury do you suspect?

V. Situations

<u>**Instructions:**</u> *Have each student work with a partner to cooperatively analyze and address the following situations.*

1. An athlete has sustained a supracondylar fracture of the left elbow region. What major complication may occur with this injury? How would you assess this condition?

2. A gymnast lost his hand position on a giant swing on the horizontal bar and fell to the floor on an outstretched arm. Immediate pain and deformity is evident along the distal forearm. How will you assess this condition to rule out injury to the neurovascular structures of the arm?

3. A wrestler has acute swelling about an inch in diameter on the proximal posterior ulna. His history reveals constant friction to the area. What condition do you suspect, what anatomical structures are involved, and how will you manage this condition?

4. A softball player, when sliding head first into second base, jammed an outstretched arm into the base. Observation reveals a noticeable posterior deformity of the elbow. The athlete is unwilling to move the elbow and is in extreme pain. Explain and demonstrate how to perform circulatory and neurological assessment of this injury. What immediate first-aid care would you render?

V. Situations (Con't)

5. After receiving a severe blow to the forearm, a lineman is having problems flexing his wrist and fingers. There is rapid swelling, discoloration, and a diminished distal pulse. Passive stretching of the wrist flexors causes increased pain. What condition do you suspect and what anatomical structures are involved with this injury?

VI. Special Tests

Instructions: *Have the students work with a partner to perform the following special tests and explain the rational for each test.*

- **Valgus stress test**
- **Common extensor tendinitis test**
- **Tinel's sign**
- **Pinch grip test**
- **Varus stress test**
- **Medial epicondylitis test**
- **Elbow flexion test for ulnar neuritis**

VII. Teaching Strategies

1. **Invite a biomechanist to class to discuss the kinematics of the throwing motion occurring at the elbow joint.**

2. **Invite an orthopedist to discuss injuries and surgical procedures associated with the throwing motion.**

3. **Invite a tennis pro to class to discuss the stresses placed on the elbow during tennis activity. Also have the tennis pro demonstrate how the racket (grip or string tightness) may affect the elbow during various tennis strokes.**

4. **Invite a brace expert to class to demonstrate the various braces used for elbow injuries during treatment and activity or debate the pros and cons of counterforce braces in the prevention and treatment of tennis elbow.**

Instructor's Key

I. Anatomy

Refer to Table 11-1 on page 421 in the text

II. Key Terms

Carrying angle — — — — The angle between the humerus and the ulna when the arm is in anatomical position

Cubital valgus — — — — — Angle of an extended elbow that deviates toward the radial side more than 20 degrees

Cubital varus — — — — — Angle of an extended elbow that deviates less than 10 degrees toward the radial side

Resting position — — — — Slightly flexed position of the elbow that allows for maximal volume to accommodate any intraarticular swelling

Volkmann's contracture — Ischemic necrosis of the forearm muscles and tissues caused by damage to the blood flow

Nightstick fracture — — — Fracture of the ulna due to a direct blow commonly seen in football players

Tackler's exostosis — — — Irritative exostosis arising from the anterior or lateral humerus

Ectopic bone — — — — — Proliferation of bone ossification in an abnormal place

Periostitis — — — — — — — Inflammation of the periosteum (outer membrane covering the bone)

Fibrositis — — — — — — — — Inflammation of fibrous tissue

Forearm splints — — — — Chronic strain to the forearm muscles

Epicondylitis — — — — — Inflammation and microrupturing of the soft tissues on the epicondyle of the distal humerus

Little leaguer's elbow — — Tension stress injury of the medial epicondyle seen in adolescents

Pronator syndrome — — — Median nerve is entrapped by the pronator teres, leading to pain on activities involving pronation

II. Key Terms (Con't)

Wrist drop ——————— Weakness and/or paralysis of the wrist and finger extensors due to damage to the radial nerve

Malaise ———————— Lethargic feeling of general discomfort; out-of-sorts feeling

III. Kinematics

Refer to Table 11-l on page 421 in the text and page 444 in the text.

Movement	Muscles	Normal ROM
Elbow flexion	Biceps brachii	140–150°
	Brachioradialis	
	Brachialis	
Elbow extension	Triceps brachii	0–10°
Forearm supination	Supinator biceps brachii	90°
Forearm pronation	Pronator quadratus	90°

IV. Simulations

1 Lateral Epicondylitis (Tennis Elbow)

(Refer to pages 433–436 in the text)

During palpations, did the students palpate the following structures for point tenderness, swelling, deformity, skin temperature, sensation, or other signs of trauma? Did they compare bilaterally?

- olecranon process
- radius
- ulna
- lateral epicondyle region
- proximal attachment of wrist extensor and supinator muscle groups

1A. During special tests, did the students:

- perform active, passive, and resistive elbow flexion, extension, forearm supination and pronation, and wrist extension and flexion
- pay particular attention to manual resistance of wrist extension and supination, noting pain or tenderness near the lateral epicondyle
- ask the individual to squeeze each hand, comparing grip strength
- perform all tests bilaterally

Did the treatment protocol include ice, compression, elevation, anti-inflammatories, decrease in activities that aggravate the condition, and medical referral dependent on the degree of injury? (Refer to Field Strategy 11-5 on text page 437 for management protocol)

2 Contusion with Secondary Myositis Ossificans

(Refer to pages 425–430 in the text)

Did the students observe bilaterally for:

- swelling, discoloration, deformity, or other signs of trauma

Did the students palpate bilaterally for:

- point tenderness, swelling, deformity, skin temperature, sensation, or other signs of trauma

2A. Did the students suspect a contusion from the repetitive blocking activity of the football player? Since palpation revealed a hardend mass of soft tissue, did the students suspect development of myositis ossificans? Treatment involves standard acute injury care and referral to a physician.

3 Medial Epicondylitis "Little Leaguer's Elbow"

Refer to Field Strategy 11-4 on page 435 in the text.

During the history, did the students determine if the injury was chronic or acute? Did they ask:

- when, where, and how questions
- about throwing technique and training regimen (increase or decrease in throwing)
- what phase of the throwing motion pain occurs
- any previous injury, treatment, and medications
- the type of pain (dull, sharp, radiating, constant, intermittent, localized, general, increased during activity)
- ask if rest relieves symptoms

3A. Did the students palpate the following structures bilaterally for point tenderness, swelling, deformity, sensation, skin temperature, or other signs of trauma?

- medial epicondyle
- origin of wrist flexors and pronators
- ulna
- olecranon
- ulnar nerve
- radius

During special tests, did the students perform the following bilaterally?
- active, passive, and resisted elbow flexion, extension, forearm pronation and supination, and wrist extension and flexion
- pay particular attention to manual resistance of wrist flexion and pronation noting pain or tenderness near the medial epicondyle
- ask the athlete to squeeze each hand, comparing grip strength
- perform Tinel's sign for ulnar nerve involvement

Did the students determine that the ulnar nerve may be associated with this injury?
Did the students suspect medial epicondylitis or little leaguer's elbow?

V. Situations

1. Volkmann's Contracture - (Refer to page 439 in the text) - A major complication that results from a supracondylar fracture is Volkmann's contracture. Did the students do the following to assess this condition?
- determine if the brachial artery or median nerve was damaged secondary to the fracture by looking and feeling for coldness, whiteness, or numbness in the hand of the affected arm
- perform passive extension of the fingers on the affected arm, noting increasing pain and aggravation to the injury

2. Forearm Fracture - Refer to Field Strategy 11-6 on page 441 in the text - To rule out injury to neurovascular structures of the forearm secondary to the forearm fracture, did the students perform the following bilaterally:
- palpate for a distal radial or ulnar pulse
- check for sensation distal to the injury (See Figure 11-22 on page 448 in text)
- check for skin color and skin temperature distal to the injury

3. Olecranon Bursitis - (Refer to page 430 in the text)
- Did the students identify this injury as olecranon bursitis?
- Did management include applying ice, compression, elevation, and other standard acute care procedures?

V. Situations (Con't)

4. Posterior Elbow Dislocation - (Refer to Field Strategy 11-2 on page 432 in the text) - To perform neurological and circulatory assessment for this injury, did the students perform the following bilaterally?

- check for a distal pulse
- check for sensation distal to the injury
- check for skin color and skin temperature distal to the injury

Did the students perform the following immediate first-aid care:

- immobilize the limb in the position found
- treat for shock
- immediately refer to a physician or call 9ll for assistance

5. Compartment Syndrome - (Refer to page 438 in the text)
Did the students suspect a possible compartment syndrome?
Did the students determine that the following structures may be involved with this injury?

- wrist and finger flexors of the anterior compartment
- median nerve

VI. Special Tests

Refer to pages 444 to 450 in the text.

Chapter 12 Wrist and Hand Injuries

After completing this chapter the student should be able to:

- **Locate the important bony and soft tissue structures of the wrist and hand**
- **Describe the motions of the wrist and hand and identify the muscles that produce them**
- **Explain what forces produce the loading patterns responsible for common injuries of the wrist and hand**
- **Recognize and manage common injuries to the wrist and hand**
- **Demonstrate a thorough assessment of the wrist and hand**
- **Demonstrate general rehabilitation exercises for the wrist and hand**

I. Anatomy Review

Materials Needed:
SKELETON ANATOMICAL WRIST AND HAND CHARTS NONPERMANENT MARKERS

Instructions: *Divide the students into pairs and have them:*
- identify the following anatomical structures on the skeleton or anatomical charts
- palpate and draw the anatomical structures on their partner using the nonpermanent marker.

Bony and Ligamentous Structures of the Wrist

-radius
-ulna
-styloid process of ulna
-scaphoid or navicular
-lunate
-triquetrum
-pisiform
-trapezium
-trapezoid
-capitate
-hamate
-volar radiocarpal ligament
-dorsal radiocarpal ligament
-radial collateral ligament
-ulnar collateral ligament

Bony and Ligamentous Structures of the Hand and Fingers

-carpometacarpal joint
-intermetacarpal joint
-metacarpophalangeal joint
-interphalangeal joint
-metacarpal bones 1-5
-phalanges 1-5
-ulnar and radial collateral ligaments of thumb and phalanges

Muscles of the Wrist and Hand

-extensor pollicis longus
-extensor pollicis brevis
-flexor pollicis longus
-abductor pollicis longus
-extensor indicis
-extensor digitorum
-extensor digiti minimi
-flexor digitorum profundus
-flexor digitorum superficialis
-flexor pollicis brevis
-abductor pollicis brevis
-opponens pollicis
-adductor pollicis
-abductor digiti minimi
-flexor digiti minimi brevis
-opponens digiti minimi
-dorsal interossei
-palmar interossei
-lumbricales

Nerves and Blood Vessels of the Wrist and Hand

-median nerve
-ulnar nerve
-radial nerves
-radial artery
-ulnar artery
-digital arteries

II. Key Terms

__Instructions:__ *Instruct the students to define the following terms.*

Volar
Dorsal
Saddle joint
Extrinsic muscles
Intrinsic muscles
Brachial plexus
Circumduction
Aseptic necrosis
Anatomical snuff box
Hypothenar
Thenar
Boxer's fracture
Bennett's fracture
Gamekeeper's thumb
Coach's finger
Jersey finger
Mallet finger
Boutonniere deformity
Trigger finger
de Quervain's tenosynovitis
Ganglion cyst
Subungual hematoma
Paronychia
Felon
Osteomyelitis
Carpal tunnel syndrome
Cyclist's palsy
Bowler's thumb

III. Kinematics of the Wrist and Hand

Instructions: *Divide the students into pairs and have them perform the following with one student being the athlete and the other being the athletic trainer.*

Have the athlete perform the following movements while the athletic trainer names the muscles that are performing the movements along with the normal range of motion for each movement. **(Refer to pages 459–462 and 484 in the text)**

- forearm pronation and supination
- wrist flexion and extension
- radial deviation
- ulnar deviation
- finger flexion and extension
- finger abduction and adduction
- thumb flexion, extension, abduction, and adduction
- opposition of the thumb and little finger

Now that the students have determined range of motion of the wrist and hand through subjective means, have them measure wrist and finger flexion with the use of a goniometer.

IV. Simulations

Instructions: *Divide the students into groups of three with one student the injured athlete, another the athletic trainer, and the third an observer. Have the students exchange roles from simulation to simulation.*

1 **A cheerleader is complaining of pain over the right anatomical snuff box. Complete a history and observation of this injury.**

1A. You have determined that the cheerleader fell on an outstretched hand yesterday during the execution of a back flip. Observation reveals minor swelling but no discoloration or deformity. Palpation reveals sharp pain in the anatomical snuff box. What injury should be suspected? How will you manage this injury?

2 **The goalie on the soccer team reports a history of a hyperextension type injury to the ring finger of the right hand. Explain and demonstrate observation and palpation for this injury.**

2A. Observation reveals minor swelling, some discoloration, but no deformity. Palpation produces point tenderness around the proximal phalanx that increases with compression and percussion along the long axis of the extended finger. You suspect a possible phalangeal fracture. Explain and demonstrate how to splint this type of fracture.

3 **A gymnast is experiencing pain during vaulting and floor routines when the body weight is supported on the hands. Explain and demonstrate how to determine the difference between a wrist fracture and wrist sprain.**

3A. All fracture tests are negative, and you believe the injury is a wrist sprain due to excessive extension. How will you manage this condition? Can the individual continue to practice with some support provided to prevent the injury from getting worse?

4 **While holding a jersey tightly in one hand in an effort to stop the opposing player, a rugby player felt a sharp pain in the ring finger. Through observation and special tests, explain and demonstrate how to determine the differences between jersey finger and mallet finger. Identify what anatomical structures are involved with each injury.**

4A. The observation and special tests conclude that the rugby player has ruptured the flexor digitorium profundus tendon of the injured finger. Explain and demonstrate the first-aid care for this injury.

V. Situations

__Instructions:__ *Have each student work with a partner to cooperatively analyze and address the following situations.*

1. A softball catcher was hit in the throwing hand by the bat of the hitter. Observation reveals immediate swelling over the fifth metacarpal of the affected hand. Explain and demonstrate how to determine a possible fracture, and then demonstrate how to properly immobilize the region and apply standard first-aid procedures.

2. A track athlete hit a hurdle and fell onto the cinder track and now has an abrasion on the palmar side of the hand. What immediate and long-term concerns must be kept in mind in cleaning this superficial wound?

3. An offensive lineman comes off the field complaining of pain in the right thumb. Explain and demonstrate how to determine the difference between a possible navicular fracture, ligament, and muscle injury.

4. A weight lifter pinched a finger between a weight and a weight rack. Blood has accumulated under the fingernail. The fingertip is extremely painful from the increasing pressure. What factors determine whether or not it is necessary to relieve the pressure?

V. Situations (Con't)

5. A long-distance cyclist is complaining of numbness in the little finger and medial half of the ring finger and is unable to abduct the little finger on both hands. The cyclist cannot recall a single incident that could have caused this condition. The cyclist's training distance has increased significantly in the past two weeks. What possible factors could be involved in this condition? What suggestions can be offered to help alleviate the symptoms yet allow the cyclist to continue training?

VI. Special Tests

Instructions: *Have the students work with a partner to explain and demonstrate the following special tests:*

-Phalen's test **-Tinel's sign** **-Froment's sign**

VII. Teaching Strategies

1. Invite an occupational therapist to demonstrate the various types of splints used for injuries to the wrist, hand, and fingers. Also have them discuss rehabilitation techniques and exercises.

2. Invite an orthopedic hand specialist to discuss the types of injuries and surgical procedures used for injuries to the wrist, hand, and fingers.

3. Invite a gerontologist to discuss arthritic conditions often seen in the wrist, hand, and fingers of the elderly, and the implications arthritis may have on rehabilitation.

4. Divide the students into pairs and have them practice the various types of taping and bracing techniques used for wrist, hand, and finger injuries.

Instructor's Key

I. Anatomy

Refer to Table 12-1 on pages 459–460 in the text.

II. Key Terms

Anatomical snuff box — — Region directly over the scaphoid bone bounded by the extensor pollicis brevis medially and the extensor pollicis longus laterally

Aseptic necrosis — — — — The death or decay of tissue due to a poor blood supply

Bennett's fracture — — — Fracture-dislocation to the proximal end of the first metacarpal at the carpal-metacarpal joint

Bowler's thumb — — — — Compression of the digital nerve on the medial aspect of the thumb, leading to paresthesia in the thumb

Boutonniere deformity — — Rupture of the central slip of the extensor tendon at the middle phalanx, resulting in no active extensor mechanism at the PIP joint

Boxer's fracture — — — — Fracture of the fifth metacarpal resulting in a flexion deformity due to rotation of the head of the metacarpal over the neck

Brachial plexus — — — — Nerve plexus formed by the intertwined ventral rami of the lower four cervical and first thoracic nerves (C_5-T_1)

Carpal tunnel syndrome —— Compression of the median nerve as it passes through the carpal tunnel, leading to pain and tingling in the hand

Circumduction — — — — Circular motion of a body segment, resulting from sequential flexion, abduction, extension, and adduction, or vice versa

Coach's finger — — — — — Fixed flexion deformity of the finger, resulting from dislocation at the PIP joint

Colles' fracture — — — — Fracture involving a dorsally angulated and displaced, and a radially angulated and displaced fracture within one and one-half inches of the wrist

II. Key Terms (Con't)

Cyclist's palsy — — — —	Seen when biker's lean on the handlebar an extended period of time, resulting in paresthesia in the ulnar nerve distribution
de Quervain's tenosynovitis-	An inflammatory stenosing tenosynovitis of the abductor pollicis longus and extensor pollicis brevis tendons
Dorsal — — — — — — — —	Referring to the back of the hand
Extrinsic muscles — — —	Muscles with the proximal attachment located outside of the part it moves or acts upon
Felon — — — — — — — — —	Abscess within the fat pad of the fingertip
Galeazzi's fracture — — —	Radial fracture with an associated dislocation of the ulna at the distal radial ulnar joint
Ganglion cyst — — — — —	Benign tumor mass commonly seen on the dorsal aspect of the wrist
Hypothenar — — — — — —	Mass of intrinsic muscles of the little finger, including the abductor digiti minimi, flexor digiti minimi brevis, and opponens digiti minimi
Intrinsic muscles — — — —	Muscles with the proximal and distal attachments located within the body part it moves or acts upon
Jersey finger — — — — —	Rupture of the flexor digitorum profundus tendon from the distal phalanx due to rapid extension of the finger while actively flexed
Mallet finger — — — — —	Rupture of the extensor tendon from the distal phalanx due to forceful flexion of the phalanx
Monteggia's fracture — —	Ulnar fracture with an associated dislocation of the radial head
Osteomyelitis — — — — —	Inflammation or infection of the bone and bone marrow
Paronychia — — — — — —	Infection along the nail fold commonly associated with a hangnail
Saddle joint — — — — —	Joint at which one bone surface has a concave saddle-like shape and the articulating bone surface is reciprocally shaped

II. Key Terms (Con't)

Smith's fracture — — — — Forearm fracture with volar angulation or displacement; opposite of Colles' fracture

Stenosing — — — — — — — Narrowing of an opening or stricture of a canal; stenosis

Subungual hematoma — — Collection of blood under the fingernail caused by direct trauma

Thenar — — — — — — — — Mass of intrinsic muscles of the thumb, including the flexor pollicis brevis, abductor pollicis brevis, and opponens pollicis

Trigger finger — — — — — — Condition whereby the finger flexors contract but are unable to reextend because of a nodule within the tendon sheath or the sheath being too constricted to allow free motion

Volar — — — — — — — — — Referring to the palm of the hand

III. Kinematics of the Wrist and Hand

Refer to Table 12-1 on pages 459–460 in the text and to page 484 in the text.

Motion	Muscles	Range of Motion
Wrist flexion	Flexor carpi radialis	80–90°
	Flexor carpi ulnaris	
	Palmaris longus	
Wrist extension	Extensor carpi radialis longus	70–90°
	Extensor carpi radialis brevis	
	Extensor carpi ulnaris	
Radial deviation	Flexor carpi radialis	15°
	Extensor carpi radialis	
Ulnar deviation	Flexor carpi ulnaris	30–45°
	Extensor carpi ulnaris	

IV. Simulations

1 Scaphoid

Refer to pages 477–478 in the text

During the history, did the students ask:
- where, when, and how questions
- if the injury was acute or chronic
- about the type of pain the individual is experiencing (dull, sharp, radiating, constant, intermittent, localized, general, increased during activity)
- ask about previous injuries, treatment, or medications.

(Refer to Field Strategy 12-3 on text page 481)

During observations, did the students observe bilaterally for:
- swelling, discoloration, deformity, and other signs of trauma
- the shape, contour, and posture of the hand
- surgical scars or incisions

Did the students palpate bilaterally for:
- swelling, temperature, deformity, point tenderness
- other signs of trauma

1A. Did the students suspect a fracture to the scaphoid because of point tenderness over the anatomical snuff box?

2 Phalangeal Fracture

Did the students observe bilaterally for swelling, deformity, discoloration, or other signs of trauma?

Did the students palpate bilaterally for point tenderness, swelling, crepitation, deformity, sensation, and circulation?

2A. Did the students immobilize the injured finger in 30 degrees of flexion to reduce the pull of the flexor tendon?

3 Wrist Sprain

(Refer to Field Strategies 12-3 on page 481 in the text and 12-4 on page 483 in the text).

To determine a possible wrist fracture, did the students:

- determine the mechanism of injury in the history
- palpate for point tenderness and crepitus over the bones and observe for any deformity
- ask the individual to perform active range of motion to determine willingness and physiological functioning of the region
- perform compression, distraction, and percussion tests for a possible fracture

If fracture tests were negative, did the students apply resisted range of motion exercises to determine a possible wrist sprain?

3A. Did the students manage the wrist sprain with:

- ice, compression, elevation,
- progressive range of motion and strength exercises
- supportive taping or bracing

4 Jersey Finger

(Refer to page 469 in the text)

Did the students observe bilaterally for:

- swelling, deformity, discoloration, and other signs of trauma
- deformity of the distal attachment of the flexor profundus tendon
- the functioning of the flexor profundus tendon by asking the individual to actively flex the PIP joint while keeping the distal interphalangeal joint (DIP) extended

Mallet Finger

- observe for deformity of the distal attachment of the extensor tendon
- test the function of the extensor tendon by asking the individual to actively extend the DIP joint of the effected finger

4A. Did the students immobilize the affected finger, apply ice, and refer the person to a physician?

V. Situations

1. Metacarpal Fracture - (Refer to Field Strategy 12-2 on page 479 in the text) -
To determine if the injury is a possible fracture, did the students:

- perform a history to determine the mechanism of injury
- observe for swelling, discoloration, deformity, or bone protrusions
- palpate for deformity, crepitation, and point tenderness over the metacarpal area
- apply compression and percussion through the axis of the fifth metacarpal, noting increased pain

To care for this injury, did the students:

- immobilize the hand in a relaxed fist position, apply ice, and refer to a physician

2. Abrasion - Immediate concerns for this abrasion injury include:

- preventing HIV or hepatitis B virus (HBV) by using universal precautions (Refer to pages 61 and 464 in text)
- cleansing the wound thoroughly to prevent infection
- applying sterile nonadherent dressing

Long-term concerns for this abrasion may include:

- checking the wound daily for signs of infection
- referring the individual to a physician if infection is noted

3. Thumb Injury - Did the students determine that:

- a scaphoid fracture would produce pain over the anatomical snuff box and increase with radial deviation and wrist extension
- to test a ligament injury to the thumb, a valgus or varus stress test is applied to determine laxity of the ligaments if no fracture is suspected
- to determine a muscle injury, active and resistive range of motion can be applied to the thumb musculature

4. Subungual Hematoma - (Refer to Field Strategy 12-1 on page 473 in the text) - Did the students determine that the athlete has a subungual hematoma? Did they decide that if it is not absolutely necessary to relieve the pressure from under the nail, they should not do so because this opens an avenue for infection? If pressure must be relieved, the procedure should be carried out under the direction of a physician.

V. Situations (Con't)

5. Cyclist's Palsy - (Refer to text page 475 to 476) - Did the students determine the condition to be cyclist's palsy and that factors related to this condition include:

- leaning on the handlebar for extended period of time
- not switching hand positions frequently
- improper fit of the bike to the rider

Did the students offer the following suggestions to help alleviate the symptoms so that the cyclist could continue training:

- padding the handlebars
- wearing padded gloves
- varying hand positions
- getting properly fitted for the bike

VI. Special Tests

Refer to pages 483 to 489 in the text

Chapter 13 Head and Facial Injuries

After completing this chapter the student should be able to:

- **Locate the important bony and soft tissue structures of the head and facial region**
- **Identify forces responsible for common injuries to the head and facial region**
- **Recognize specific injuries to the skull and facial area**
- **Demonstrate a thorough assessment of a cerebral injury**
- **Recognize and demonstrate immediate care of facial injuries**
- **Identify protective padding and commercial products used to prevent and manage head and facial injuries**

I. Anatomy Review

Materials Needed:

SKELETON | ANATOMICAL CHARTS OF HEAD AND FACE | NONPERMANENT MARKERS

Instructions: *Divide the students into pairs and have them:*

- identify the following anatomical structures on the skeleton and anatomical charts.
- palpate and draw the anatomical structures on their partner using the nonpermanent marker.

Structures of the Head and Face

-frontal bone
-occipital bone
-sphenoid bone
-ethmoid bone
-parietal bone
-temporal bone
-maxilla
-mandible
-zygomatic arch
-nasal bone
-lacrimal
-glabella
-palatine
-temporal mandibular joint
-carotid artery
-cranial nerves

Identify the functions of the following anatomic structures:

-optic nerve
-olfactory nerve
-oculomotor and trochlear nerves
-vestibulocochlear nerve
-gray matter of cerebral cortex
-medulla oblongata
-cerebrum
-cerebellum
-lacrimal glands
-iris
-retina
-middle meningeal artery

II. Key Terms

Instructions: *Instruct the students to define the following terms.*

Dyspnea
Tinnitus
Cauliflower ear
Vertigo
Photophobia
Battle's sign
Concussion
Postconcussion syndrome
Post-traumatic memory loss
Retrograde amnesia
Diffuse injuries
Dural sinuses
Focal injuries
Meninges
Meningitis
Gray matter
White matter
Epistaxis
Malocclusion
Intruded
Extruded
Otitis media
Otitis externa
Serous otitis
Conjunctivitis
Sty
Subconjunctival hemorrhage
Tunics
Hyphema
Diplopia
Myopia
Detached retina
Nystagmus
Periorbital ecchymosis
Raccoon eyes
Contrecoup injuries
Decompression

III. Simulations and Situations

Instructions: *Divide the students into groups of three with one student being the injured athlete, another being the athletic trainer, and the third student an observer. Have the students exchange roles from simulation to simulation as they perform the following simulated experiences.*

1. A basketball player has fallen and sustained what appears to be a superficial cut on the back of the head. The cut is bleeding profusely. What anatomical structure(s) are likely to have been damaged and why? How serious is this injury likely to be? Explain and demonstrate the immediate treatment protocol.

III. Simulations and Situations (Con't)

2. A rugby player was hit in the torso region and is down on the field. During the history, you learn that the neck is sore, the player has a headache, and is also a bit dazed and dizzy. This information is confusing because you saw the injury and know that the player did not receive a blow to the head. Explain how and why the individual may be experiencing these symptoms. What other signs and symptoms should be farther investigated during the HOPS process? How would you determine when this individual should return to participation?

3. A softball player collided with the shortstop, accidentally taking an elbow to the side of the head. The individual is dizzy and has a mild headache. There is no immediate memory loss, and the pupils are normal. After 15 minutes of icing the injured area, the individual reports an increasing headache and is feeling nauseous. The player appears lethargic, disoriented, and sensitive to sunlight. What might be happening, and how will you manage this situation?

4. A swimmer during a backstroke set misjudged the distance to the wall and collided head first into the wall. After the assessment, you determine the swimmer experienced a mild concussion. What instructions are you going to give the swimmer when leaving for the day? What follow-up care will you provide?

4A. Two days after the swimmer experienced the injury, he/she reports a persistent headache and an inability to concentrate. What other questions should be asked of the swimmer about the condition? What condition may the swimmer be experiencing? What is standard protocol for managing this injury?

5. A hockey player was taking a shot on goal when the stick hit the jaw of the player who was guarding him. That player came off the ice bleeding from the mouth and unable to close the jaw. Explain and demonstrate observation and palpation of this hockey player. What type of injury do you suspect and why?

6. In fielding a softball, the third baseman was struck in the nose by the ball. Explain and demonstrate how to determine the difference between an epistaxis and possible nasal fracture through the evaluation procedures. What treatment protocol would be used for each injury?

7. A basketball player was going up for a rebound and was struck in the eye by an opposing player's finger. The eye is swollen and closed. Attempts to open the eye causes tearing and pain. Explain and demonstrate how to determine the differences between a periorbital ecchymosis, corneal abrasion, detached retina, and possible orbital fracture. Explain the treatment protocol for each condition.

IV. Special Test

Instructions: *Have the students work with a partner to perform the following special tests and explain the rationale for each test.*

- **100 minus 7 test**
- **Romberg's test**
- **Heel/toe walking**
- **Finger to nose test**
- **Stork stand**

V. Teaching Strategies

1. **Invite a panel of professionals consisting of an opthomologist, dentist, and neurologist to discuss their roles on the athletic health care team.**

2. **Invite a general practitioner to further discuss injuries of the eyes, ears, nose, and face and their treatment.**

3. **Take the students on a field trip to a nearby medical facility and ask the radiotechnical department to present how head injuries are identified through radiographic and other diagnostic means (CAT scan and MRI).**

4. **Invite a neurologist to discuss the types of head injuries most often seen in sport activities and how these injuries are treated.**

Instructor's Key

I. Anatomy

Refer to Figure 13-1 on page 498 in the text and Table 13-1 on page 501 in the text.

II. Key Terms

Dyspnea — Shortness of breath or difficulty in breathing

Tinnitus — Ringing or other noises in the ear due to trauma or disease

Cauliflower ear — Hematoma between the perichondrium and cartilage of the outer ear; auricular hematoma

Vertigo — Balance disturbance characterized by a whirling sensation of one's self or external objects

Photophobia — Abnormal sensitivity to light

Battle's sign — Delayed discoloration behind the ear due to basilar skull fracture

Concussion — Violent shaking or jarring action of the brain, resulting in immediate or transient impairment of neurological function

Postconcussion syndrome — Delayed condition characterized by persistent headaches, blurred vision, irritability, and inability to concentrate

Post-traumatic memory loss — Forgetting events after an injury

Retrograde amnesia — Forgetting events prior to an injury

Diffuse injuries — Widespread disruption to the function and/or structure of the brain

Dural sinuses — Formed by tubular separations in the inner and outer layers of the dura matter, these sinuses function as small veins for the brain

Focal injuries — Localized cerebral damage

Meninges — Three protective membranes that surround the brain and spinal cord

II. Key Terms (Con't)

Meningitis ——————— Inflammation of the meninges of the brain and spinal column

Gray matter —————— Composed of neuron cell bodies, dendrites, and short unmyelinated axons

White matter —————— Composed of myelinated nerve axons; it is the myelin sheaths that give the tissue its characteristic white coloring

Epistaxis ———————— Profuse bleeding from the nose

Malocclusion —————— Inability to bring teeth together in a normal bite

Intruded ———————— Tooth driven in an inward direction

Extruded ——————— Tooth driven in an outward direction

Otitis media —————— Localized infection in the middle ear secondary to upper respiratory infections

Otitis externa —————— Bacterial infection involving the lining of the auditory canal; swimmer's ear

Serous otitis —————— Fluid buildup behind the eardrum in association with otitis media and upper respiratory infections

Conjunctivitis —————— Bacterial infection, leading to itching, burning, watering, inflamed eye; pinkeye

Sty ——————————— Infection of the sebaceous gland of an eyelash or eyelash follicle

Subconjunctival hemorrhage– Minor capillary ruptures in the eye globe

Tunics ———————— Three layers of protective tissues that surround the eye

Hyphema ——————— Serious condition with hemorrhage into the anterior chamber of the eye

Diplopia ———————— Double vision

Myopia ———————— Nearsightedness

II. Key Terms (Con't)

Detached retina — — — — Neurosensory retina is separated from the retinal epithelium by swelling

Nystagmus — — — — — — — Abnormal jerking or involuntary eye movement

Periorbital ecchymosis — — Swelling and hemorrhage into the surrounding eye lids; black eye

Raccoon eyes — — — — — — Delayed discoloration around the eyes from anterior cranial fossa fracture

Contrecoup injuries — — — Injuries away from the actual injury site due to axial rotation and acceleration

Decompression — — — — Surgical release of pressure from fluid or blood accumulation

III. Simulations and Situations

1. Scalp Laceration - Refer to page 512 in the text - Did the students evaluate the athlete for a possible concussion? Did the students use universal precautions during their evaluation and treatment protocol? Did the students apply direct pressure to the wound, bandage, and ice? Did the students refer the basketball player to a physician for possible sutures?

2. Concussion - Refer to pages 509 to 512 and Tables 13-4 (text page 511) and 13-6 (text page 519) in the text - Did the students determine that the rugby player may have a contrecoup concussion? Did the students further evaluate the rugby player by performing a HOPS assessment for a concussion? Did the students determine if the player could return to activity according to the signs and symptoms presented, particularly to those related to consciousness and memory loss?

3. Severe Concussion/Head Injury - Did the students determine that an immediate physician referral was needed since the softball player may be experiencing signs and symptoms related to a possible epidural hematoma?

4. Postconcussion Syndrome - Did the students determine that the swimmer may be experiencing postconcussion syndrome? Did they further investigate the swimmer's condition by asking further questions related to postconcussion syndrome? Did the students refer the swimmer to a physician?

(Refer to Field Strategy 13-2 on page 518 and Table 13-6 on page 519 in the text and for further identification and treatment procedures for cranial injuries)

III. Simulations and Situations (Con't)

5. Fractured Mandible - Did the students observe the following?
- malocclusion
- deformity
- swelling
- other signs of trauma (lacerations)

Did the students palpate the following structures for point tenderness, muscle spasms, and deformity?
- maxilla
- mandible
- zygomatic
- nasal bone
- TMJ
- other related soft tissue

Did the students practice universal precautions since the individual was bleeding from the mouth?

Did the students conclude that the hockey player may have a fractured mandible? What is the treatment protocol for this injury? (Refer to text pages 519 to 520)

6. Nasal Injury - Refer to text pages 521–523 and Field Strategy 13-4 on page 524 - Did the students explain and demonstrate that a nasal fracture would indicate the following signs?
- deformity
- swelling
- crepitus in the bridge of the nasion
- ecchymosis under the eyes

Did the students stand behind and above the injured player to observe the injury? What protocol would be used for a nasal fracture and epistaxis?

III. Simulations and Situations (Con't)

7. Eye Injury - Refer to text pages 527 to 532 and Field Strategy 13-6 on page 532 - Did the students conclude that a corneal abrasion may be present because of the:

- tearing
- pain upon movement
- increased pain upon blinking of eye
- photophobia

Did the students determine that a detached retina would result in lights flashing on and off when the individual opened the eyes several days following the injury, or they might state that a blanket has covered part of the field of vision?

During the students' assessment of an orbital fracture, did they ask the athlete to look upward with both eyes and observe if the injured eye failed to do this movement?

How did the students indicate they would treat each of these eye injuries? In each case, what would determine a physician referral? (Refer to Field Strategy 13-6 on page 532 in the text)

IV. Special Tests

Refer to pages 513–516 in the text for cranial injury assessment.

Chapter 14 Injuries to the Spine

<u>After completing this chapter the student should be able to:</u>

- **Locate and explain the functional significance of the important bony and soft tissue structures of the spine**
- **Describe the motion capabilities in the different regions of the spine**
- **Explain what factors contribute to mechanical loads on the spine**
- **Specify strategies to reduce spinal stress in preventing low back pain**
- **Identify anatomical variations that may predispose individuals to spine injuries**
- **Recognize and describe common sports injuries to the spine and back**
- **Demonstrate a thorough assessment of the spine**
- **Demonstrate rehabilitative exercises for the spine**

I. Anatomy Review

<u>Materials Needed:</u>

SKELETON ANATOMICAL SPINE CHARTS NONPERMANENT MARKERS

<u>Instructions</u>: *Divide the students into pairs and have them:*
- *identify the following anatomical structures on the skeleton and anatomical charts*
- *palpate and draw the anatomical structures on their partner using the nonpermanent marker.*

Structures of the Spine

-cervical spines Cl-C7
-thoracic spines Tl-T12
-lumbar spines L1-L5
-sacral spines Sl-S5
-coccyx
-intervertebral disc
-pars articularis
-spinous and transverse process
-axis and atlas
-supraspinous ligament
-ligament flavum
-sternocleidomastoid
-trapezius
-erector spinae
-levator scapula
-occiput
-mastoid process
-lumbar curve
-cervical curve
-thoracic curve
-cauda equina

II. Key Terms

Instructions: *Instruct the students to define the following terms.*

Motion segment
Atlas
Axis
Annulus fibrous
Nucleus pulposus
Cauda equina
Reflex
Kyphosis
Lordosis
Scheuermann's disease
Scoliosis
Spondylolisthesis
Spondylolysis
Spina bifida occulata
Spinal stenosis
Neurapraxia
Burner
Wedged fracture
Osteopenia
Sciatica
Prolapsed disc
Extruded disc
Coccygodynia
Ipsilateral

III. Kinematics

Instructions: *Divide the students into pairs and have them perform the following with one student being the athlete and the other being the athletic trainer.*

1. Have your partner perform spinal flexion and extension. In what plane of movement are the motions occurring? Does maximal spinal flexion and extension occur in the lumbar, cervical, or thoracic vertebra? What is the degree of maximal spinal flexion?

2. Have your partner perform lateral flexion. In what plane of movement does this motion occur? What is the normal degree of motion for lateral flexion in the lumbar vertebra?

3. Have your partner perform spinal rotation and forward bending of the cervical vertebra. What is the average range of motion for cervical rotation and forward bending?

IV. Simulations

Instructions: *Divide the students into groups of three with one student being the injured athlete, another the athletic trainer, and the third student an observer. Have the students exchange roles from simulation to simulation as they perform the following simulated experiences.*

1 **A football player is down on the field, and you have been beckoned to render care. The individual is lying supine, the head turned to the side, and is not moving. Perform a primary assessment.**

1A. The athlete has a pulse and is breathing adequately. The individual has regained consciousness. Continue with the secondary survey and conduct a history of this injury. Would you remove the face mask on the athlete?

1 Con't

1B. During the history you discover the player is dizzy, has a mild headache, and has mild pain in the neck. Explain and demonstrate observation, palpation, and special testing procedures.

lC. After completing the on-the-field secondary survey, the player still has a mild headache, mild neck pain, and is somewhat dizzy, but complete sensory and motor function appears normal. Explain and demonstrate how to remove the player from the field. Explain and demonstrate a full off-the-field assessment for this injury.

lD. You have rechecked the player's balance, neck range of motion, vital signs, vision, memory, and have reevaluated for concussion. What criteria will determine if the player can return to competition or must be immediately transported to the hospital?

2

A defensive lineman charged the quarterback preparing to throw a pass and struck the throwing arm, forcing it into excessive external rotation, abduction, and extension. An immediate burning sensation traveled down the length of the quarterback's arm, and now his thumb is tingling. What might have happened here? Explain and demonstrate your observations and palpations. What special tests would you use?

2A. The quarterback exhibits radiating pain down his right arm into his thumb, and he has weakness in his biceps. The tingling resolves within a few minutes. What criteria are used to determine when the player can return to participation?

3

A cheerleader is complaining of an aching pain during trunk flexion aggravated with resisted hyperextension that produces sharp shooting pains into the low back and down the posterior leg. This condition has been present for four weeks and is not getting better. The individual cannot recall a traumatic episode that may have caused the condition. A physician has not been seen, nor have radiographs been taken of the lumbar region. Explain and demonstrate palpation procedures for this injury.

3A. What special tests can rule out a disc injury? What special tests can identify if the injury is nerve related? Explain and demonstrate these tests.

3B. What criteria are used to determine if the individual should be referred to a physician?

V. Situations

Instructions: *Have each student work with a partner to cooperatively analyze and answer the following situations.*

1. After practice, a wrestler is complaining of a sore neck that is most comfortable with the head in a slightly rotated position to the right. Point tenderness is present in the left sternocleidomastoid muscle and right trapezius muscle. Explain and demonstrate the special testing procedures for this injury. While doing these tests please indicate the normal range of motion for the various neck movements.

2. An adolescent butterfly stroker is complaining of localized pain and tenderness in the midback region. The pain developed gradually and only hurts during execution of the stroke. Explain and demonstrate palpations and special tests using the HOPS procedure. During the assessment, perform a scan examination. What conditions would you suspect to occur in this area of the thoracic spine?

VI. Special Tests

Instructions: *Have the students work with a partner to perform the following special tests and explain the rational for each test.*

- **Myotome testing**
- **Cervical compression test**
- **Cervical distraction test**
- **Straight leg raising test**
- **Reflex testing**
- **Prone knee bending test**
- **Sacroiliac test**

VII. Teaching Strategies

1. Have the students discuss how axial loading occurs during a hit in football when the player making the tackle uses the crown of his head as the major point of impact. Have them demonstrate the anatomical failure of the spine that results from such a force by drawing a diagrammatic representation on the board.

2. Have the students explain and demonstrate proper lifting techniques used to minimize tension within the lumbar muscles and spine.

3. Have a physical therapist demonstrate rehabilitation techniques for lumbar spine injuries.

Instructor's Key

I. Anatomy

Refer to Figures 14-1 and 14-2 in the text (pages 536–531) and Table 14-1 on text pages 541 to 542.

II. Key Terms

Motion segment ———— Two adjacent vertebrae and the intervening soft tissues; the functional unit of the spine

Atlas —————————— The first cervical vertebra; named because it supports the skull

Axis —————————— The second cervical vertebra; named after its bony prominence around which the atlas rotates

Annulus fibrous ———— Tough outer covering of the intervertebral disc composed of fibrocartilage

Nucleus pulposus ———— Gelatinous-like material comprising the inner portion of the intervertebral disc

Cauda equina ————— Lower spinal nerves that course through the lumbar spinal canal, resembling a horse's tail

Reflex ————————— Action involving stimulation of a motor neuron by a sensory neuron in the spinal cord without involvement of the brain

Kyphosis ———————— Excessive curve in the thoracic region of the spine

Lordosis ———————— Excessive curve in the lumbar region of the spine

Scheuermann's disease —— Osteochondrosis of the spine due to abnormal epiphyseal plate behavior that allows herniation of the disc into the vertebral body, giving a characteristic wedge-shaped appearance

Scoliosis ———————— Lateral rotational spinal curvature

Spondylolisthesis ———— Anterior slippage of a vertebrae, resulting from a complete bilateral fracture of the pars interarticularis

Spondylolysis —————— A stress fracture of the pars interarticularis

II. Key Terms (Con't)

Spina bifida occulata — —	Congenital defect in the vertebral canal characterized by absence of the laminae and spinous process
Spinal stenosis — — — —	A loss of cerebrospinal fluid around the spinal cord due to deformation of the spinal cord or a narrowing of the neural canal
Neurapraxia — — — — —	Injury to a nerve that results in temporary neurological deficits followed by complete recovery of function
Burner — — — — — — — —	Burning or stinging sensation characteristic of a brachial plexus injury
Wedged fracture — — — —	A crushing compression fracture that leaves a vertebra narrowed anteriorly
Osteopoenia — — — — —	Condition of reduced bone mineralization or density of a bone
Sciatica — — — — — — — —	Compression of a spinal nerve due to a herniated disc, annular tear, myogenic or muscle-related disease, spinal stenosis, facet joint arthropathy, or compression from the piriformis muscle
Prolapsed disc — — — — —	Condition when the eccentric nucleus produces a definite deformity as it works its way through the fibers of the annulus fibrous
Extruded disc — — — — —	Condition in which the nuclear material come into the spinal canal and runs the risk of impinging adjacent nerve roots
Coccygodynia — — — — —	Prolonged or chronic pain in the coccygeal region due to irritation of the coccygeal nerve plexus
Ipsilateral — — — — — — —	Situated on, pertaining to, or affecting the same side, as opposed to contralateral

III. Kinematics

Cervical Spine
(Refer to pages 542 to 544 and Table 14-2 (text page 544)

IV. Simulations

1 Head/Neck Down on the Field

Refer to pages 566 to 570 in the text

During the primary assessment, did the students:

- check for consciousness by shouting the athlete's name?
- check for pulse by palpating the carotid artery?
- check for breathing by palpating or watching the chest rise and fall
- check the pupils for size and responsiveness
- An athlete's pulse rate will range from 40 to 80 beats per minute
- An athlete's respiration rate will range from 10 to 15 breaths per minute
- Pupils should be equal and constrict with light and dilate with no light

1A. Did the students remove the face mask before starting the history? It is recommended that you remove the face mask even though the athlete is breath ing with no difficulty. Why? This is a safety measure in case the athlete stops breathing during the assessment. Without the face mask, rescue breathing and CPR is much easier.

During the history, did the students ask the athlete about the following?

- headache
- diplopia
- blurred vision
- feeling in legs and arms
- tinnitus
- nausea
- what happened
- what hurts
- retrograde amnesia questions
- post-traumatic amnesia questions
- logic and recall questions
- previous injury to the head or neck

1 Head/Neck Down on the Field (Con't)

1B. During the observation, did the students observe for the following?

-bleeding or fluid from ears, nose, mouth
-bumps, deformities, other signs of trauma
-the athlete's body position
-discoloration, swelling
-skin color
-pupil size

During palpation, did the students palpate:

- the neck for bumps, deformities, and point tenderness
- sensory function of the brachial plexus and sacral plexus bilaterally
- motor function of the brachial plexus and sacral plexus bilaterally
- injuries to other parts of the body other than head or neck

1C. Before removing the athlete from the field, did the students have the athlete sit up slowly, asking about increased dizziness or headache? Did they use the two-person assistance procedure to get the athlete off the field?

With the athlete on the sideline, did the students continue the assessment by:

- having the athlete sit and recheck vitals including pupillary reaction to light
- reasking questions about headache, dizziness, nausea, memory, blurred vision, tinnitus, sensory, and motor functions
- repalpating the neck and checking for range of motion
- check balance by using Romberg' test, sobriety test, and finger to nose test

1D. After completing the assessment, the students found that the athlete had a mild headache and sore neck. Did the students decide that since the athlete was never unconscious that he could return to the game if he becomes asymptomatic?

2 Brachial Plexus Injury

(Refer to pages 557 to 558 in text)

During the observation of the quarterback's arm, did the students observe for:

- swelling, deformity, discoloration, other signs of trauma
- the body position of the athlete and how he was treating his injury
- skin color

2 Brachial Plexus Injury (Con't)

During palpation, did the students palpate for:
- swelling, deformity
- point tenderness of the neck and shoulder region
- sensory function of the brachial plexus nerves
- motor function of the brachial plexus nerves

During the special tests, did the students:
- check range of motion for the neck and shoulder region
- check strength of the brachial plexus myotomes, particularly the biceps, deltoid, and external rotators
- check grip strength

2A. Did the students determine that if the athlete has no related neck or shoulder injury that he could return to the game if strength of the biceps return to normal?

3 Lumbar Spine Injury

(Refer to Tables 14-4 on page 562, 14-5 on page 564, and 14-8 on page 574 in the text)

During palpation, did the students palpate for:
- swelling, muscle spasms, point tenderness, deformities, other trauma
- bony structures, soft tissue, muscles

3A. During special tests, did the students use the straight leg test to determine nerve root involvement or sciatica? Did the students use the valsalva test to determine disc injury? Did they check the Achilles tendon reflex?

3B. Did the students determine that if the athlete had signs of nerve root involvement or disc injury that a referral to a physician is warranted?

V. Situations

1. Neck Strain - Refer to page 556 and Figures 14-24 A to D on text pages 572–573 - During the testing procedures, did the students have the athlete
- perform forward bending, looking for 80 degrees of flexion
- perform backward bending, looking for 90 degrees of extension
- perform sidebending, looking for 45 degrees of bending
- perform rotation, looking for 90 degrees of rotation

V. Situations (Con't)

Did the students have the athlete perform these movements both actively and against manual resistance?

2. Thoracic Spine Injury - Did the students palpate the following structures for point tenderness, deformity, muscle spasms, swelling, and temperature during their assessment?
- thoracic spinous processes
- intervertebral ligaments
- intervertebral muscles
- latissimus dorsi

Did the students perform the following special tests?
- forward bending and extension
- lateral bending and rotation
- deep breathing
- shoulder flexion, extension, abduction, adduction, horizontal flexion, and extension
- movements of the butterfly stroke

Did the students determine that since the swimmer was an adolescent and that the movement associated with the butterfly stroke caused pain that the swimmer may have Scheuermann's disease?

VI. Special Tests

Refer to pages 571 to 578 in the text.

Chapter 15 Throat, Thorax and Visceral Injuries

<u>After completing this chapter the student should be able to:</u>

- **Locate the important bony and soft tissue structures of the throat, thorax, and viscera**
- **Recognize specific injuries of the throat, thorax, and viscera**
- **Describe the life-threatening conditions that can occur spontaneously or as a result of direct trauma to the throat, thorax, and viscera**
- **Demonstrate an assessment of the throat, thorax, and visceral regions**
- **Describe the pelvic/abdominal stabilization exercises and abdominal strengthening exercises**

I. Anatomy Review

<u>Materials Needed:</u>

SKELETON — ANATOMICAL CHARTS OF THE THROAT, THORAX, AND VISCERAL REGIONS

NONPERMANENT MARKERS

<u>Instructions</u>: *Divide the students into pairs and have them:*

- *identify the following anatomical structures on the skeleton or anatomical charts*
- *palpate and draw the anatomical structures on their partner (where appropriate) using the nonpermanent marker.*

Structures of the Throat

-pharynx
-larynx
-trachea
-esophagus
-carotid arteries
-superior thyroid artery
-facial artery
-lingual artery
-subclavian artery
-costocervical artery
-thyrocervical trunk artery
-vertebral artery

Structures of the Thorax

- -thoracic cage (sternum, ribs, costal cartilage, thoracic vertebrae)
- -pleura
- -bronchial tubes
- -heart
- -pectoralis minor
- -serratus anterior
- -subclavius
- -levator scapulae
- -trapezius
- -rhomboids
- -external intercostals
- -internal intercostals
- -diaphragm

Structures of the Visceral Region

- -spleen
- -liver
- -pancreas
- -kidneys
- -adrenal glands
- -stomach
- -small and large intestines
- -bladder
- -ureter
- -appendix
- -gallbladder
- -sacrum
- -ischium
- -pubis
- -ilium
- -aorta
- -left and right coronary arteries
- -left and right common carotid arteries
- -brachial arteries
- -intercostal arteries
- -renal arteries
- -splenic artery
- -hepatic artery
- -rectus abdominis
- -external oblique
- -internal oblique
- -transverse abdominous
- -quadratus lumborum
- -inguinal ligament
- -linea alba

II. Key Terms

Instructions: *Instruct the students to define the following terms.*

Alveoli
Pulmonary circuit
Systemic circuit
Atria
Ventricles
Vocal cords
Atrioventricular valves
Semilunar valves
Chyme
Peristalsis
Hepatitis
Cirrhosis
Laryngospasm
Flail chest
Runner's nipple
Cyclist's nipple
Gynecomastia
Stitch-in-side
Hyperventilation
Pulmonary contusion
Subcutaneous emphysema
Pneumothorax
Tension pneumothorax
Traumatic asphyxia
Hemothorax
Arrhythmia
Sudden death
Marfan's syndrome
Athletic heart syndrome
Solar plexus punch
Hernia
Peritonitis
Infectious mononucleosis
Kehr's sign
Appendicitis
McBurney's point
Hematuria
Proteinuria

III. Simulations

Instructions: *Divide the students into groups of three with one student being the injured athlete, another being the athletic trainer, and the third student an observer. Have the students exchange roles from simulation to simulation as they perform the following simulated experiences.*

1 **A cyclist was riding over loose gravel on the road when the rear tire skidded sideways causing the rider to fall. During the fall, the rider fell forward onto the handlebars. The rider is complaining of pain on the right lower side of the rib cage. Explain and demonstrate palpations and special testing procedures for this injury.**

1A. Palpation reveals point tenderness over the lower right rib cage. There is no deformity or crepitation noted. However, during coughing and deep breaths, the cyclist experiences severe pain in the injured area. Manual lateral compression of the rib cage also increases the intensity of pain. What injury do you suspect and how will you manage this injury?

2 **A football defensive back was making a tackle with his right arm extended. He reports feeling a snapping sensation over his right upper chest wall and complains of an aching fatigue like pain. Explain what factors should be observed in this injury.**

2A. Observation reveals swelling and ecchymosis to the anterior right chest wall. Deformity is noted medially to the chest wall. Continue the evaluation with special testing.

2B. Shoulder motion is limited by pain during range of motion, and horizontal adduction and internal rotation are weak. What may be present?

3 **A second baseman fielded a base hit and threw the ball to first base. By accident, the ball struck a base runner going to second base directly on the sternum. The runner immediately collapsed on the base path. You arrived at the scene to find the player in obvious pain and gasping for air. How will you manage this situation? What would indicate the need for EMS?**

3A. What underlying serious problems do you need to be concerned about during the treatment of this injury?

4 **A colleague was playing flag football when a sudden back hyperextension injury caused sharp pain in the abdominal region. There is marked tenderness and muscle guarding slightly below and to the right of the umbilicus. No swelling or discoloration is visible, nor is there radiating pain. Explain and demonstrate palpation and stress test.**

4A. During the special tests, the individual complains of pain in the abdominal area during back extension and during a modified sit-up activity. What injury do you suspect?

5 **A 20-year-old football player was struck in the abdomen with a helmet and experienced a sudden onset of abdominal pain in the upper left quadrant. Complete a history and palpate the appropriate structures for this injury.**

5A. During the history, the individual states that he is experiencing radiating pain into his upper chest and left shoulder. He feels weak and lightheaded. Blood pressure is 96/72 and his pulse is weak at 96 beats per minute. Palpation reveals point tenderness and rigidity over the upper left quadrant. What injury do you suspect, and what is your immediate first-aid procedure?

IV. Situations

<u>Instructions</u>: *Have each student work with a partner to cooperatively analyze and answer the following situations.*

1. An ice hockey player was checked into the sideboard. The opponent's elbow inadvertently struck the player's anterior neck. The player is now on the ice coughing and having difficulty swallowing. How will you control the situation and manage the injury?

2. A female runner is complaining of breast soreness. After evaluation, you have determined that she may need to purchase a sport bra. Discuss the types of sport bras available and the factors that limit motion and irritation to the breasts.

3. After a long layoff, a cross-country runner complains of a stitch in the side during the initial practice. What advice can you provide to this runner to help alleviate the pain that occurs during running?

4. After running wind sprints, the center on the basketball team is having trouble catching her breath. During the history, she reports that she feels numbness in her lips and hands, is somewhat dizzy, and has a dry mouth. What condition do you suspect, and how will you manage this condition?

IV. Situations (Con't)

5. Marfan's syndrome is a disorder most often associated with individuals who have long tubular bones. You have been asked to screen a basketball team for Marfan's syndrome. Please determine the types of screening procedures used to accomplish this task.

6. A running back has received a severe blow to the abdomen. The athlete is experiencing dyspnea. You suspect a solar plexus contusion. How will you manage this injury?

V. Teaching Strategies

1. Invite an internist to discuss anatomy and injuries to the abdomen and thorax regions.

2. Take the class on a field trip to a nearby hospital and visit the cardiology department. Have a cardiologist explain and demonstrate how EKGs and other cardiology pathology are diagnosed and treated.

3. Invite an ear, nose, and throat specialist to further discuss trauma and illness associated with athletic participation to this region of the body.

Instructor's Key

I. Anatomy

Refer to Table 15-1 on page 592 in the text.

II. Key Terms

Alveoli — — — — — — — — Air sacs at the terminal ends of the bronchial tree where oxygen and carbon dioxide are exchanged between the lungs and surrounding capillaries

Pulmonary circuit — — — Blood vessels that transport unoxygenated blood to the lungs from the right heart ventricle and oxygenated blood from the lungs to the left atrium

Systemic circuit — — — — Blood vessels that transport unoxygenated blood to the right heart atrium and oxygenated blood from the left heart ventricle

Atria — — — — — — — — — Two superior chambers of the heart that pump blood into the ventricles

Ventricles — — — — — — — Two inferior chambers of the heart that pump blood out of the heart, one to the pulmonary circuit and one to the systemic circuit

Vocal cords — — — — — — — Bands of elastic connective tissue encased in mucosal folds that enable the voice to make sound

Atrioventricular valves —— Heart valves that prevent the backflow of blood from the ventricles to the atria

Semilunar valves — — — — Heart valves that prevent the backflow of blood from the pulmonary artery and aorta to the ventricles

Chyme — — — — — — — — Paste-like substance into which food is churned in the stomach

Peristalsis — — — — — — — Periodic waves of smooth muscle contraction that propel food through the digestive system

Hepatitis — — — — — — — — Inflammation of the liver

Cirrhosis — — — — — — — — Progressive inflammation of the liver usually caused by alcoholism

II. Key Terms (Con't)

Laryngospasm	Spasmodic closure of the glottic aperture, leading to shortness of breath, coughing, cyanosis, and even loss of consciousness
Flail chest	Three or more consecutive ribs on the same side of the chest wall that are fractured in at least two separate locations
Runner's nipple	Nipple irritation due to friction as the shirt rubs over the nipples
Cyclist's nipple	Nipple irritation due to the combined effects of perspiration and windchill producing cold, painful nipples
Gynecomastia	Excessive development of the male mammary glands
Stitch-in-side	A sharp pain or spasm in the chest wall, usually on the lower right side, that occurs during exertion
Hyperventilation	Respiratory condition where too much carbon dioxide is exhaled, leading to an inability to catch one's breath
Pulmonary contusion	Contusion to the lungs due to compressive force
Subcutaneous emphysema	Presence of air or gas in subcutaneous tissue, characterized by a crackling sensation on palpation
Pneumothorax	Condition whereby air is trapped in the pleural space, causing a portion of a lung to collapse
Tension pneumothorax	Condition in which air continuously leaks into the pleural space, causing the mediastinum to displace to the opposite side and compresses the uninjured lung and thoracic aorta
Traumatic asphyxia	Condition involving extravasation of blood into the skin and conjunctivae due to sudden increase in venous pressure
Hemothorax	Condition involving the loss of blood into the pleural cavity, but outside the lung
Arrhythmia	Disturbance in heartbeat rhythm
Sudden death	Nontraumatic, unexpected death occurring instantaneously or within minutes of an abrupt change in an individual's previous clinical state

II. Key Terms (Con't)

Marfan's syndrome — — — Inherited connective tissue disorder affecting many organs, but commonly resulting in the dilation and weakening of the thoracic aorta

Athletic heart syndrome — Benign condition associated with physiological alterations in the heart

Solar plexus punch — — — A blow to the abdomen that results in an immediate inability to breathe freely

Hernia — — — — — — — — Protrusion of abdominal viscera through a weakened portion of the abdominal wall

Peritonitis — — — — — — — Inflammation of the peritoneum that lines the abdomen

Infectious mononucleosis — Viral condition caused by the Epstein-Barr virus that attacks the respiratory system and leaves the spleen enlarged and weak

Kehr's sign — — — — — — — Referred pain into the left shoulder due to a ruptured spleen

Appendicitis — — — — — — Inflammation of the appendix

McBurney's point — — — A site one-third the distance between the ASIS and umbilicus that, with deep palpation, produces rebound tenderness indicating appendicitis

Hematuria — — — — — — — Blood and red blood cells in the urine

Proteinuria — — — — — — — Abnormal concentrations of protein in the urine

III. Simulations

1 Rib Fracture

(Refer to text pages 602 to 604 and Field Strategy 15-2 on page 603)

During palpation, did the students palpate bilaterally for:

- point tenderness
- crepitation
- deformity
- spasm
- rebound pain

1 Rib Fracture (Con't)

During special tests, did the students:

- have the athlete cough and take deep breaths, noting if pain or other symptoms were associated with the injured area?
- apply manual lateral compression to the rib cage, testing for possible rib fracture?
- perform range of motion testing for the trunk, noting increased pain during lateral flexion away from the injured area?

1A. Did the students suspect the cyclist may have a rib fracture?

- Did the students apply ice to minimize pain and inflammation, immobilize the area, and refer the individual to a physician?

2 Rupture of the Pectoralis Major Muscle

(Refer to page 601 in the text)

During observation, did the students observe bilaterally for:

- swelling
- eccyhmosis
- deformity
- other signs of trauma

2A. During special tests, did the students do the following bilaterally, noting limits in range of motion, muscular weakness, and motions that increase pain?

- active, passive, and resistive range of motion of the shoulder in flexion/extension, abduction/adduction, internal/external rotation, horizontal adduction/abduction
- functional movements

2B. Did the students suspect the defensive back ruptured the right pectoralis major muscle?

3 Respiratory Distress

The runner is in obvious respiratory distress. During the management of this injury, did the students:

- initiate a primary survey
- talk to the athlete to calm them down
- assess breathing and circulation
- take vital signs
- treat for shock

3 Respiratory Distress (Con't)

Did the students indicate that EMS would be needed if:
- respirations did not return to normal
- cardiac irregularities were present

3A. Did the students determine that the impact of the ball may have caused:
- hyperventilation
- fractured sternum
- internal complications to the heart or lungs

4 Rectus Abdominus Muscle Strain

During special tests, did the students have the individual perform the following, noting limits in range motion, weakness, and increased pain?
- active, passive, and resistive trunk flexion/extension, lateral flexion, and rotation
- modified sit-ups

4A. Because pain increases with active contraction of the abdominal muscles during a modified sit-up, did the students suspect this injury was a strain to the rectus abdominus or obliques?

5 Ruptured Spleen

Refer to Table 15-5 on page 611 and Field Strategies 15-3, 15-4, 15-5, and 15-6 on text pages 611, 614, 616, and 620, respectively.

During the history, did the students:
- ask where, when, and how questions
- ask about the type of pain the athlete is experiencing
- ask if the athlete was experiencing any dizziness, nausea, weakness, numbness, or other unusual feelings

Did the students check blood pressure and pulse rate?

Did the students palpate the upper left quadrant for:
- point tenderness
- swelling
- deformity
- rebound pain
- spasms and rigidity

Did the students palpate the remaining abdomen?

5A. Did the students suspect the football player may have ruptured the spleen? Did the treatment protocol include treating for shock and immediately summoning EMS?

IV. Situations

1. Anterior Throat Trauma - (Refer to Field Strategy 15-1 on page 599 in the text) - To care for the injured hockey player, did the students reassure the individual and attempt to place the chin in a forward position to straighten the airway? Did the students make note that if breathing does not return to normal within a few minutes EMS should be summoned?

2. Sport Bra Selection - (Refer to Chapter 6, Protective Equipment, in the text, on pages 196–197 and 199)

3. Stitch in the Side - To alleviate the pain, the runner can:
- forcibly exhale through pursed lips
- breathe deeply and regularly
- lean away from the affected side
- stretch the arm on the affected side over the head as high as possible

4. Hyperventilation - Did the students suspect the basketball player is experiencing hyperventilation? Did the management plan include:
- calm the player down
- have the player concentrate on slow inhalations through the nose and exhaling through the mouth to slow breathing
- breathe into a paper bag

5. Marfan's Syndrome Screening - (Refer to pages 606–607 and Table 15-4 on text page 607) - Did the students include the following screening procedures for Marfan's syndrome?
- height and arm span measurements
- past history of rheumatic fever, hypertension, cardiac problems, or chronic disease
- symptoms of syncope, near syncope, palpitations, low exercise tolerance, chest discomfort on exertion, or dyspnea
- family history of syncope, hypertension, premature coronary disease, or sudden death
- measurements of blood pressure and pulse, auscultation of the heart for cardiac rhythm, murmurs, and abnormal heart sounds, and palpation of peripheral pulses

IV. Situations (Con't)

6. Solar Plexus Contusion - Did the students manage the solar plexus contusion by:
- assessing airway for obstruction
- removing any mouthguard or dental apparatus
- loosening restrictive clothing and/or equipment around the abdomen
- having the individual flex his knees toward his chest
- summoning EMS if breathing does not return to normal within a few minutes

Chapter 16 Conditions Related to the Reproductive System

After completing this chapter the student should be able to:

- **List the primary and accessory organs in the female and male reproductive system**
- **Explain the signs and symptoms of common injuries to the female and male genitalia**
- **Describe management of injuries to the female and male genitalia**
- **Indicate the mode of transmission, signs and symptoms, and current treatment of sexually transmitted diseases.**
- **Identify the various menstrual irregularities and the implications they may have on sport participation**
- **Describe how sport performance may be affected by the use of oral contraceptives and IUDs**
- **Specify indications and contraindications for sport participation during pregnancy**

I. Anatomy Review

Materials Needed:

SKELETON — ANATOMICAL CHARTS

Instructions: *Divide the students into pairs and have them identify the following anatomical structures on the skeleton or anatomical charts and explain the function of each structure.*

Anatomy of the Genitalia

-ovaries
-testes
-fallopian tubes
-uterus
-vagina
-vulva
-epididymis
-ductus deferens
-seminal vesicles
-prostate gland
-bulbourethral gland
-scrotum
-penis
-pelvic girdle

II. Key Terms

Instructions: *Have the students define the following key terms.*

Primary sex organs
Accessory sex organs
Steroids
Menses
Estrogens
Progesterone
Androgens
Hydrocele
Varicocele
Hematocele
Pruritus
Retroviruses
Dysmenorrhea
Oligomenorrhea
Amenorrhea
Osteopenia

III. Simulations

Instructions: *Divide the students into groups of three with one student being the injured athlete, another the athletic trainer, and the third student an observer. Have the students exchange roles from simulation to simulation as they perform the following experiences.*

1 **A soccer player was struck in the groin by a knee. He was not wearing a protective cup and immediately fell to the ground. What possible conditions can occur as a result of direct trauma to the male genitalia?**

1A. The soccer player has sustained injury to the testicles and they are in spasm. Explain and demonstrate how to manage the condition. What signs and symptoms would indicate referral to a physician is necessary?

2 **A basketball player is complaining of painful urination and has open sores on the penis. What might you suspect, and how will you address your concerns with the athlete? What advice will you provide to the athlete?**

2A. The basketball player has been diagnosed with a sexually transmitted disease. He has been warned to avoid sexual contact with anyone until his next appointment with the physician. What can be done in the work environment to prevent the spread of sexually transmitted diseases?

3 **After watching a softball player for the past 3 weeks, you suspect she may have hepatitis. She appears lethargic, easily tires, and has notable signs of yellowing in the whites of her eyes. What clues in the history would confirm your suspicions?**

3A. After referring the softball player to the physician, your hunch was confirmed, and she was diagnosed with hepatitis. What type of treatment will the player need to follow?

IV. Situations

Instructions: *Have each student work with a partner to cooperatively analyze and answer the following situations.*

1. A cyclist is complaining of transient paresthesia of his penis when riding for long periods of time. What condition might you suspect? What anatomical structure is involved, and what preventative measures can prevent this condition from recurring?

2. A baseball team has been struck with an outbreak of tinea cruris. You have been asked to educate the team on prevention and then discuss treatment for this condition.

3. A lean 16-year-old distance runner has reported she has not had a menstrual period in 3 months and is concerned that she may be pregnant. What other menstrual irregularities could account for this absence of menses?

4. A female gymnast is experiencing dysmenorrhea and is having difficulty getting through practice because of the discomfort. Indicate how you would treat this woman for this condition.

5. A female athlete wants to begin taking oral contraceptives for birth control reasons. What implications may these oral contraceptives have on her performance, and what adverse effects might she experience? Please discuss these with the athlete.

6. A recreational runner has asked for information concerning running and exercise during pregnancy. What advice can you provide?

V. Teaching Strategies

1. **Invite a gynecologist to discuss the various types of sexually transmitted diseases and specific concerns to a sport participant.**
2. **Invite a dermatologist to discuss the various types of skin conditions that affect the genital region and their treatment.**
3. **Develop role play exercises for the students concerning how they would deal with an athlete who: 1) has been tested positive for HIV; 2) premenstrual syndrome; 3) has herpes; and 4) is pregnant.**
4. **Have the students write a paper concerning sexually transmitted diseases and debate if athletes are more or less at risk for these diseases.**
5. **Have the students discuss the development and complications associated with osteoporosis.**
6. **Have the students observe in the athletic training room and determine if universal safety precautions are being followed.**

Instructor's Key

I. Anatomy

Refer to Figures 16-1 and 16-2 on page 628 in the text.

II. Key Terms

Primary sex organs ———	Reproductive organs responsible for producing gametes (ovum and sperm)
Accessory sex organs ——	Organs that transport, protect, and nourish gametes
Steroids ————————	A large family of chemical substances including endocrine secretions and hormones
Menses —————————	Phase in the menstrual cycle when the thickened vascular walls of the uterus, the unfertilized ova, and blood from damaged vessels are lost during the menstrual flow
Estrogens ———————	A class of hormones that produce female secondary sex characteristics and affect the menstrual cycle
Progesterone —————	Hormone responsible for thickening the uterine lining in preparation for the fertilized ovum
Androgens ———————	A class of hormones that promote development of male genitals and secondary sex characteristics and influence sexual motivation
Hydrocele ———————	Swelling in the tunica vaginalis of the testes
Varicocele ———————	Abnormal dilation of the veins of the spermatic cord leading to engorgement of blood into the spermatic cord veins during a standing position
Hematocele ———————	A rapid accumulation of blood and fluid in the scrotum around the testicle and cord
Pruritus ————————	Intense itching
Retroviruses ——————	Any virus of the family Retroviridae known to reverse the usual order of reproduction within the cells they infect
Dysmenorrhea ————	Difficult or painful menstruation; menstrual cramps

II. Key Terms (Con't)

Oligomenorrhea — — — — Infrequent menstrual cycles

Amenorrhea — — — — — Absence or abnormal cessation of menstruation

Osteopenia — — — — — — Decreased calcification or density of bone

III. Simulations

1 Testicular Spasm

Did the students determine that the following conditions could result from direct trauma to the male genitalia?

- contusion to the testes or penis
- scrotal hemorrhage
- hydrocele
- hematocele
- tunica vaginitis

1A. In the students' management plan for the injury, did they:

- instruct the individual to bring his knees to his chest to relieve the spasms
- apply cold compresses to reduce swelling and hemorrhage
- treat for shock if needed
- encourage the individual to do periodic self assessment

Did the students conclude that the following signs and symptoms would indicate referral to a physician?

- swelling of testicles
- severe discoloration
- increase pain and discomfort

2 Sexually Transmitted Disease

(Refer to Table 16-1 on pages 635–637 and Field Strategy 16-2 on text page 640)

Did the students suspect a sexually transmitted disease such as herpes or gonorrhea? Did the students approach the individual with a caring and sensitive attitude, suggesting the individual seek medical attention as soon as possible and refrain from any sexual contact until after the appointment?

2A. Did the students suggest following OSHA standards governing exposure to blood-borne pathogens to prevent the spread of these diseases in the work environment?

3 Hepatitis

During the history, did the students identify the following factors to suggest the individual may have hepatitis?

- yellowing of eyes
- mild flu-like symptoms
- poor appetite
- nausea
- dizziness
- general muscle aches
- fatigue and headaches
- abdominal pain

3A. Did the students include the following as part of the treatment protocol for hepatitis?

- bed rest
- plenty of fluids

IV. Situations

l. Biker's Penis - Did the students determine that the cyclist was experiencing biker's penis as a result of pressure to the pudendal nerve? Did the students suggest the following measures to prevent this condition from recurring?

- adjusting the height and tilt of the saddle
- adjusting the number of cycling bouts
- standing up on the pedals periodically to relieve the pressure on the affected nerve

2. Tinea Cruris - (Refer to Field Strategy 16-l on text page 634) - Did the preventive measures include:

- proper drying after showers
- wearing cotton briefs and shorts
- wearing nonrestrictive shorts and briefs
- keeping the area dry with powders

Did the treatment protocol include:

- application of antifungal agents such as Micatin, Lotrimin, Mycelex, or Tinactin twice daily for at least 1 month
- keeping the area clean and dry
- wearing absorbent clothing such as those made from cotton
- if the condition does not clear, refer to a physician

IV. Situations (Con't)

3. Menstrual Irregularities - Other than pregnancy, did the students suggest that the distance runner could also be experiencing secondary amenorrhea and should be seen by a physician to rule out pregnancy?

4. Dysmenorrhea - Was the following suggested for treating the dysmenorrhea?
- over-the-counter medications such as Midol, Advil, or Ibuprofen to relieve the pain and cramping
- eating a diet high in fiber and fluid and low in salt to decrease the risk of dysmenorrhea

5. Oral Contraceptives - (Refer to text pages 643–644) - Did the students suggest that oral contraceptives can increase the risk for certain conditions but that low-dose oral contraceptives and regular exercise can offset many of the risks, providing a safe, effective birth control method for active women.

6. Exercise During Pregnancy - (Refer to Field Strategy 16-3 on page 646 and Table 16-6 on page 647 in the text) - Did the students determine that exercise problems of pregnant women include:
- poor balance
- overheating and dehydration
- leg, hip, or abdominal pain
- avoiding weight-loading activities such as volleyball, basketball, or horseback riding
- avoiding ballistic activity and doing no impact aerobics
- weight training with lightweight and high repetitions
- decreasing running distance and intensity as pregnancy progresses
- consult a physician before starting or continuing any exercise program

Chapter 17 Other Health Conditions Related to Sports

After completing this chapter the student should be able to:

- **Identify what impact environmental conditions, such as altitude and poor air quality, have on sport participation**
- **Describe the signs, symptoms, and management of common respiratory tract infections**
- **Describe the signs, symptoms, and management of common disorders of the gastrointestinal tract**
- **Explain the physiological factors involved in diabetes and differentiate the management of diabetic coma from insulin shock**
- **Identify common contagious viral diseases**
- **Describe the signs and management of an individual experiencing an epileptic seizure**
- **List common substances abused by athletes and the impact on the individual's health and sport performance**
- **Describe the various eating disorders and explain guidelines for safe weight loss and weight gain**

I. Key Terms

Instructions: *Instruct the students to define the following terms.*

Hypoxia
Rhinitis
Rhinorrhea
Malaise
Sinusitis
Pharyngitis
Influenza
Hay fever
Bronchitis
Infectious mononucleosis
Asthma
Bronchospasm
Gastroenteritis
Diarrhea
Constipation
Hemorrhoids
Diabetes
Hyperglycemia
Hypoglycemia
Epilepsy
Clonic state
Tonic state
Hypertension
Anemia
Sickle cell anemia
Infarcts
Therapeutic drugs
Antipyretic
Neoplasm
Bulimia
Anorexia nervosa

II. Simulations

Instructions: *Divide the students into groups of three with one student being the injured or sick athlete, another being the athletic trainer, and the third student serving as an observer. Have the students exchange roles from simulation to simulation as they perform the following simulated experiences.*

1 **A volleyball player has suddenly developed a headache, general body aches, and is slightly chilled. To determine if the individual is developing the flu, what other questions would you ask, and what observations might confirm your suspicions? Demonstrate how to determine if this individual has a fever.**

1A. After doing a more thorough history and observation, you have determined that the volleyball player may indeed be experiencing flu-like symptoms. How would you manage this condition?

2 **A soccer player has been running up and down the field during full contact practice. After a few minutes, the individual begins to experience tightness in the chest, shortness of breath, and wheezing. Complete a history on this sport participant.**

2A. You have discovered that the individual has a past history of these episodes and is an asthmatic. What condition is occurring, and what is your immediate treatment protocol?

3 **A diabetic basketball player is halfway through a practice session when suddenly the player feels weak and faint. Explain and demonstrate how to determine if this player is experiencing insulin shock.**

3A. Observations and palpations reveal the individual has pale, cold, and clammy skin and shallow respirations. The individual is perspiring profusely. Explain and demonstrate how to manage this condition.

4 **A middle-aged female endurance runner is complaining of chronic fatigue and malaise, particularly when running. She appears somewhat pale and tired, but otherwise is fine. Complete a medical history of the condition.**

4A. During the history, the runner reports that she tends to have a heavy menstrual flow and does not eat meat or take iron supplements. What condition might you suspect, and how will you manage this runner?

5 **A 16-year-old football player returned from summer vacation 30 pounds heavier and able to bench press 50 additional pounds. Although he reported that he was on an aggressive weight training program over the summer, you question how these gains were made in such a short period of time. How would you further question this athlete about his increased strength gains?**

5A. After talking with the football player, you suspect he has been taking some sort of tissue-enhancing drug during his summer weight training program. Discuss with the athlete the implications these drugs may have on his health and performance. What follow-up discussions might you have with him?

6 **A baseball player reports to you complaining of inner gum pain. Please perform an observation for this complaint.**

6A. You observed white patches on the gums and stained teeth. When asked if the baseball athlete uses smokeless tobacco, he answers yes. Discuss the health implications of smokeless tobacco with this athlete.

7 **There are rumors that a swimmer was seen eating a large amount of food and then disappeared to the restroom to vomit. After returning from the restroom, her eyes appear bloodshot and she looks pale. There is also rumor that she uses diuretics; however, weight appears normal. What other signs and symptoms would you look for in this athlete that might indicate an eating disorder? Do these rumors need to be addressed? If yes, how will you address them?**

7A. After addressing these issues with the athlete, she denies having a dysfunctional eating disorder. What is your next plan of action?

7B. To prevent other swimmers from dysfunctional eating behavior, you have been asked to talk with the team about the proper weight loss that will not affect their performance. Discuss the type of information you would provide in your meeting with the swimmers.

III. Situations

Instructions: *Have each student work with a partner to cooperatively analyze and answer the following situations.*

1. A 37-year-old male with asthma is seeking advice about how to improve his cardiovascular endurance. What activities might you recommend and what guidelines should be followed in developing the exercise program?

III. Situations (Con't)

2. It is in the spring of the year, and the pollen index is high. A hurdler on the track team reports to practice with itchy and watery eyes. During the warm-up running session, the individual experiences difficulty in breathing and becomes congested. What condition do you suspect, and how would you manage this condition?

3. A male distance runner has reported the consistent need to stop and have a bowel movement while training. Is this normal for runners? What can be done about it?

4. A football player has been having bouts of diarrhea. What type of precautionary measures must be taken if this athlete is going to participate?

5. A tennis player has been diagnosed as a diabetic. The diabetes does not preclude activity or competition. Discuss how to prevent hypoglycemia episodes during exercise.

6. During warm-up, a softball player suddenly gets a glassy stare on the face, begins to smack the lips, and walks aimlessly around the field as if intoxicated. You have determined that the athlete has not been drinking or taking any medications. What condition might this individual have, and how will you manage this situation?

7. A college wrestler wants to lose weight quickly. You have heard that he may be taking diuretics to aid him in his weight loss. Discuss the problems associated with health and performance from taking diuretics as weight loss agents.

8. An athlete has suffered a severe knee injury. You have applied ice, compression, and elevation. You would like to recommend the individual take something for the pain. What type of over-the-counter medication might you recommend and why?

9. During twice a day practices in August, a good number of football players decided to go out and drink during a day off. The next day in practice there were bouts of muscle cramping, and the athletes were just not as sharp with their motor skills as in previous practices. What may have contributed to the decreases in motor skill performance and increased muscle cramping and why?

10. The track and field team is competing in 3 weeks at nationals in Denver, Colorado. Because of the high altitude, what can be done to reduce the impact of altitude on the athletes' performance?

IV. Teaching Strategies

1. Invite a pharmacologist to discuss the various over-the-counter and prescription medications used for athletic injuries and illness.

2. Instruct students on how to use a physicians' desk reference and then give them different drugs to reference in the manual.

3. Invite a substance abuse specialist to further discuss the types of drugs being used in society, especially those in your region of the country.

4. Invite a general physician or the team physician to discuss special conditions affecting the sport participant and how treatment may or may not be different for the athletic population (diabetes, asthma, common cold, flu, bronchitis, allergies)

5. Have the student prepare guidelines for athletes who want to lose weight or maintain their current weight.

6. Do a role-playing exercise where the students demonstrate how they would deal with an athlete who is: 1) anorexic; 2) alcoholic; 3) using anabolic steroids or human growth hormone; or 4) amphetamines.

7. Invite a professional counselor to discuss issues concerning the athletic trainer's role in the intervention and care of participants who are: 1) anorexic or bulemic; 2) alcoholic; 3) using tissue-enhancing substances; or 4) using illegal substances.

8. Have the students write a one- or two-page paper on why sport participants may be more susceptible to conditions of the respiratory tract.

9. Have the students discuss or write a paper about why athletes may or may not be more at risk for the use of alcohol and other drugs.

Instructor's Key

I. Key Terms

Hypoxia — — — — — — — — Reduction of oxygen supply to tissue despite adequate blood flow

Rhinitis — — — — — — — — Inflammation of the nasal membranes with excessive mucus production, resulting in nasal congestion and postnasal drip

Rhinorrhea — — — — — — — Clear nasal discharge

Malaise — — — — — — — — General discomfort; feeling out-of-sorts

Sinusitis — — — — — — — — Inflammation of the paranasal sinuses

Pharyngitis — — — — — — Viral, bacterial, or fungal infection of the pharynx, leading to a sore throat

Influenza — — — — — — — Acute infectious respiratory tract condition characterized by malaise, headache, dry cough, and general muscle aches

Hay fever — — — — — — — Seasonal allergic rhinitis caused by air borne pollens and/or fungus spores

Bronchitis — — — — — — — Inflammation of the mucosal lining of the tracheobronchial tree characterized by bronchial swelling, mucus secretions, and dysfunction of the cilia

Infectious mononucleosis — Acute viral disease caused by the Epstein-Barr virus manifested by malaise and fatigue

Asthma — — — — — — — — Disease of the lungs characterized by constriction of the bronchial muscles, increased bronchial secretions, and mucosa swelling, all leading to airway narrowing and inadequate airflow during respiration

Bronchospasm — — — — — — Contraction of the smooth muscles of the bronchial tubes causing narrowing of the airway

Gastroenteritis — — — — — Inflammation of the mucous membrane of the stomach or small intestine

I. Key Terms (Con't)

Diarrhea	Loose or watery stool, resulting when food residue rushes through the large intestine before there is sufficient time to absorb the remaining water
Constipation	Infrequent or incomplete bowel movements
Hemorrhoids	Dilations of the venous plexus surrounding the rectal and anal area that can become exposed if they protrude internally or externally
Diabetes	Metabolic disorder characterized by near or absolute lack of the hormone insulin, or insulin resistance, or both
Hyperglycemia	Abnormally high levels of glucose in the circulating blood that can lead to diabetic coma
Hypoglycemia	Abnormally low levels of glucose in the circulating blood that can lead to insulin shock
Epilepsy	Disorder of the brain characterized by recurrent episodes of sudden, excessive discharges of electrical activity in the brain
Clonic state	Movement marked by repetitive muscle contractions and relaxation in rapid succession
Tonic state	Steady rigid muscle contractions with no relaxation
Hypertension	Sustained elevated blood pressure above the norms of 140 mm Hg systolic or 90 mm Hg diastolic
Anemia	Abnormal reduction in red blood cell volume or hemoglobin concentration
Sickle cell anemia	Abnormalities in hemoglobin structure, resulting in a characteristic sickle- or crescent-shaped red blood cell that is fragile and unable to transport oxygen
Infarcts	Clumping together of cells that block small blood vessels, leading to vascular occlusion, ischemia, and necrosis in organs
Therapeutic drugs	Prescribed or over-the-counter medications used to treat an injury or illness

I. Key Terms (Con't)

Antipyretic ——————— Medication used to bring a fever down

Neoplasm ——————— Mass of tissue that grows more rapidly than normal and may be either benign or malignant

Bulimia ———————— Personality disorder manifested by episodic bouts of binging large amounts of food followed by purging and feelings of guilt, self-disgust, and depression

Anorexia nervosa ——— Personality disorder manifested by extreme aversion toward food, resulting in extreme weight loss, amenorrhea, and other physical disorders

II. Simulations

1 Flu and Common Cold

The volleyball player had a headache and body aches. Did the students ask if the player had or was experiencing:

- chills
- malaise
- general muscle soreness
- a hacking cough
- sore throat

Did the students observe for:

- watery eyes
- fatigue
- pale skin

Did the students measure the body temperature by using an oral thermometer? Is this the most accurate way to measure core temperature?

1A. Did the management include:

- rest
- plenty of fluids
- cough medication
- NSAIDS
- physician referral

2 Exercise-Induced Asthma

During the history, did the students:

- determine if the athlete needed emergency medical attention by checking the athlete's vital signs
- ask if the athlete had ever experienced these symptoms before
- ask if the athlete had allergies
- ask if the athlete had asthma
- ask if the athlete had been sick recently with an upper respiratory infection

2A. Did the students suspect the soccer player may be experiencing exercise-induced asthma?

Did the management plan include:

- a physician referral
- making sure the player adheres to inhalers that the physician may prescribe
- making sure the player has a progressive warm-up prior to exercise and a cool-down period postexercise

(Refer to Field Strategy 17-2 on text page 656 for exercise strategies for individuals with asthma)

3 Diabetic Athlete...Insulin Shock

Did the students observe for:

- signs of dizziness
- aggressive behavior
- intense hunger
- pale, cold, clammy skin
- profuse sweating
- fainting

Did the students palpate for:

- skin temperature
- vital signs

3A. Did the management plan include:

- getting sugar into the individual quickly by placing sugar under the tongue
- physician referral

(Refer to Field Strategies 17-4 on text page 661 and 17-5 on text page 662)

4 Anemia

Did the students ask:

- if the individual has been sick
- if the individual has eaten that day and what was eaten
- if she is currently menstruating and how heavy is the flow
- if she is taking any iron supplements

4A. Did the students suspect iron-deficiency anemia in the distance runner based on her age, distance running, and heavy menstrual flow?

Did the management plan include referral to a physician to rule out other underlying conditions?

5 Steroids

Did the students' questions include:

- what type of diet the individual was on during the weight training program
- what type of weight training program he was involved with
- if the individual was experiencing any mood swings, depression, or violent behavior

(Refer to Table 17-5 on text page 671)

5A. Did the students approach the athlete in a nonthreatening manner, showing care and concern? Did they educate the athlete about the negative effects associated with steroid and other tissue-enhancing drug use? Did they suggest the athlete visit with a physician or counselor?

6 Smokeless Tobacco Use

Did the students observe:

- periodontal bone loss
- tooth loss
- gum irritation
- white patches on the gums
- stained teeth

6A. During the discussion about health implications of smokeless tobacco use, did the students include:

- bad breath
- decreased taste perception
- periodontal bone loss
- tooth loss
- nicotine addiction
- oral infections and cancer

7 Bulimia

Did the students include the following signs and symptoms during their evaluation?

- depression
- low self-esteem
- gastrointestinal irritation
- irregular menses
- Russell's sign
- chipmunk face

(Refer to Tables 17-9 on text page 677 and 17-10 on text page 679)

Did the students conclude that the rumors need to be addressed and that they should approach the individual in a non threatening manner? Did the discussion include:

- a caring and concerned attitude
- short- and long-term health effects and the effects on sport performance
- encourage the individual to seek professional counseling
- physician referral

7A. Did the students' plan of action include:

- continued support for the individual
- observation of the individual
- monitoring vital signs and other health-related measures
- continued encouragement to seek counseling

***The students must remember not to be an enabler for the bulimic athlete.**

7B. Refer to Tables 17-9 on text page 677; 17-10 on text page 679; 17-11 on text page 680; and Field Strategy 17-7 on text page 670.

III. Situations

1. Asthma and Exercise - Did the students' exercise protocol include:

- consultation with a physician
- prescription medication
- progressive warm-up and cool-down
- exercising in a warm, humid environment
- avoiding exposure to air pollutants and allergens

(Refer to Field Strategy 17-2 on page 656 in the text)

2. Allergens - Did the students suspect the hurdler had allergies? Did the management plan include:

- reducing exposure to the allergen or irritant
- suppressive medication to alleviate symptoms
- hypersensitization to reduce responsiveness to unavoidable allergens

III. Situations (Con't)

3. Irregular Bowl Function - Did the students determine that irregular bowl function is not uncommon? Did they suggest the following for treatment of this condition:
- eating a high-fiber diet
- an increase in daily exercise and fluid intake
- over-the-counter medication as recommended by a physician
- if the condition continues referral to a physician is needed

(Refer to Table 17-1 on text page 657)

4. Diarrhea - Did the students include the following precautionary measures for the football player to participate?
- eating a low-fiber diet 24 to 36 hours prior to competition
- taking advantage of the morning gastrocolic reflex
- improving hydration
- taking either Pepto-Bismol, Imodium, or Lomotil for short durations

5. Hypoglycemia Prevention - Did the students include the following to prevent hypoglycemia in the tennis player?
- eat a meal 1 to 3 hours prior to activity
- exercise at the same time each day
- administer insulin more than 1 hour prior to activity
- measure blood glucose levels prior to activity
- consume additional carbohydrate foods every 30 to 45 minutes during activity
- drink plenty of fluids

(Refer to Field Strategy 17-5 on text page 662)

6. Complex Partial Seizure - Did the students determine that the softball player might be experiencing a complex partial seizure? Did the management plan include:
- looking for a medic alert tag on the individual
- not restricting the individual but helping the person into a supine position
- clear others from around the individual
- refer to physician

(Refer to Field Strategy 17-6 on page 664 in the text)

7. Diuretics - Did the students discuss the following adverse affects of using diuretics with the wrestler?
- lower plasma and blood levels
- depletion of glycogen stores which means decreased energy
- increased electrolyte loss
- impairment of body temperature regulation which increases heat illness
- lower aerobic capacity
- reduction of muscular strength and work performance

III. Situations (Con't)

8. Pain Medication - Did the students determine that as long as the individual is not allergic to acetaminophen or ibuprofen, he/she could take these over-the-counter medications safely? The individual should not be given aspirin because it prevents the clotting of blood for up to 7 days. If in doubt about the type of medication to suggest, a physician should be consulted. (Refer to Table 17-4 on pages 667–668 in the text)

9. Alcohol - Did the students determine that the following could have been related to the decreased motor skill performance and muscle cramping after a night of drinking?

- alcohol acts as a dehydrant which could lead to muscle cramping
- alcohol can negatively affect alertness, reaction time, judgment, hand-eye coordination, accuracy, and balance up to 48 hours after drinking

(Refer to Table 17-6 on page 673 in the text)

10. Altitude and Performance - Did the students suggest that the following can decrease the effects of high altitude on the track and field team?

- arrive 3 days prior to competition
- get plenty of rest
- drink plenty of fluids
- eat a diet high in carbohydrates

Chapter Test Questions

Chapter 1
Sports Injury Management and the Athletic Trainer

<u>c</u> 1. Which of the following professionals is usually not a member of the primary sports medicine team?
a. Athletic trainer
b. Coach
c. Physical therapist
d. Primary physician

<u>d</u> 2. Which of the following professionals should be available to provide immediate support to the primary sports medicine team?
a. Strength coach
b. Nutritionist
c. Equipment manager
d. Dentist

<u>a</u> 3. The National Athletic Trainers' Association predicts that nearly ____% of all interscholastic athletes will be injured each year.
a. 25
b. 35
c. 45
d. 55

<u>d</u> 4. The team physician should be primarily responsible for conducting all of these tasks except:
a. Review preseason physical exams
b. Review immunization records
c. Dispensing medications
d. Doing safety checks of equipment and facilities

<u>a</u> 5. Which of the following individuals would not typically serve as a team physician?
a. Dentist
b. Internist
c. Osteopath
d. Pediatrician

<u>c</u> 6. Which of the following tasks should not be performed by an athletic trainer?
a. Evaluation of an injury
b. Treatment of an injury
c. Diagnosis of an injury
d. Recognition of an injury

<u>d</u> 7. Evaluating an injury depends on a strong background in:
a. Human anatomy and physiology
b. Joint biomechanics
c. Tissue healing and repair
d. All of the above

<u>d</u> 8. Therapeutic agents that enhance tissue healing while reducing pain and disability are called:
a. Antigens
b. Antipruritics
c. Antiseptics
d. Modalities

<u>c</u> 9. The individual responsible for administering and supervising recreational sport activities or activity areas is called a(n):
a. Athletic trainer
b. Coach
c. Sport supervisor
d. Athletic director

<u>a</u> 10. Ethical responsibilities that guide one's actions and promote high standards of conduct are called:
a. Standards of professional practice
b. Torts
c. Administrative standards
d. Standards of protocols

c 11. The organization that certifies athletic trainers is the:
a. American Medical Association
b. Athletic Trainers' of America
c. National Athletic Trainers' Association
d. American College of Sports Medicine

a 12. Which of the following is not a requirement to become an athletic trainer?
a. Proof of graduation from an accredited college with a curriculum program
b. Proof of current first aid and CPR
c. At least 25% of all clinical hours with high-risk sports
d. Endorsement of the application by a certified athletic trainer

b 13. Continuing education programs primarily provide an opportunity to:
a. Move up on the pay scale
b. Learn about innovative skills and techniques
c. Get more involved in the national organization
d. Meet old friends

c 14. Which of the following events would not qualify for continuing education units?
a. Attending workshops and seminars
b. Speaking at a symposium
c. Supervising student athletic trainers
d. Taking a correspondence or postgraduate course

d 15. A wrong done by an individual whereby the injured party seeks a remedy for damages suffered is called a:
a. Malfeasance
b. Misfeasance
c. Nonfeasance
d. Tort

b 16. Standard of care is defined as:
a. Committing an act that is not your responsibility to perform
b. Committing an act that another minimally competent professional would do in the same circumstance
c. Committing an act that is your responsibility to perform, but you use the wrong procedure
d. Failing to perform your legal duty of care

a 17. Malfeasance is defined as:
a. Committing an act that is not your responsibility to perform
b. Committing an act that another minimally competent professional would do in the same circumstance
c. Committing an act that is your responsibility to perform, but you use the wrong procedure
d. Failing to perform your legal duty of care.

a 18. A condition whereby danger is apparent, or should have been apparent, resulting in an unreasonable unsafe condition is called:
a. Foreseeability of harm
b. Misfeasance
c. Nonfeasance
d. Contributory negligence

a 19. A written guarantee that a product is safe for use is called a(n):

a. Expressed warranty
b. Implied warranty
c. Product safety standard
d. Seal test standard

d 20. According to the NATA Professional Education Committee report, most undergraduate athletic trainers are finding employment in which setting?

a. Colleges
b. High schools
c. Professional sports
d. Sports medicine clinics

Short Answer. List examples of four functions or tasks that can be performed in each of the six domains of athletic training.

Injury Prevention

1.
2.
3.
4.

Recognition and Evaluation of Injuries and Illnesses

1.
2.
3.
4.

Injury Management, Treatment, and Disposition

1.
2.
3.
4.

Injury Rehabilitation

1.
2.
3.
4.

Organization and Administration

1.
2.
3.
4.

Education and Counseling

1.
2.
3.
4.

List four factors that must be documented to prove negligence.

1.
2.
3.
4.

List five actions that can lead to litigation.

1.
2.
3.
4.
5.

ESSAY 1. Discuss the advantages and disadvantages of working in a traditional athletic training setting.

ESSAY 2. Discuss what steps can be taken at a sport facility to reduce the risk of injury.

ESSAY 3. What information should be included on a injury-reporting form.

Chapter 2
The Mechanics of Tissue Injury and Healing

b 1. What two potential effects occur when a force acts on an object?
a. Acceleration and deceleration
b. Acceleration and deformation
c. Deceleration and deformation
d. Compression and tension

a 2. What two factors determine whether an injury occurs when a force is sustained by tissues in the human body?
a. Magnitude of force and tissue's material properties
b. Compression of force and yield point of tissues
c. Tensile force and girth of tissues
d. Size of force and girth of tissues

a 3. When a structure is stronger in resisting force from certain directions than from others, it is said to be:
a. Anisotropic
b. Bilateral
c. Diastolic
d. Elastic

a 4. A force acting along the long axis of a structure is called a(n):
a. Axial force
b. Compressive force
c. Shear force
d. Tensile force

d 5. A pulling force that tends to stretch the object to which it is applied is called a(n):
a. Bending force
b. Compressive force
c. Shear force
d. Tensile force

c 6. A force that acts parallel or tangent to a plane passing through the object is called a(n):
a. Bending force
b. Compressive force
c. Shear force
d. Tensile force

d 7. The distribution of force over a given area is called:
a. Axial loading
b. Force's moment arm
c. Strain
d. Stress

d 8. The application of torque about the long axis of a structure such as a long bone can cause:
a. Axial loading
b. Bending
c. Strain
d. Torsion

b 9. Collagen fibers are relatively:
a. Easily injured
b. Inelastic
c. Inflexible
d. Weak

d 10. The fiber arrangement of the dermis enables the tissue to resist loads from:
a. Compression
b. Shear
c. Tension
d. All of the above

a 11. A strong, flat, sheet-like tissue that attaches muscles to other muscles or to bones is called a(n):
a. Aponeurosis
b. Fascia
c. Ligament
d. Tendon

c 12. The ability of a muscle to stretch is called:
a. Contractibility
b. Elasticity
c. Extensibility
d. Tensibility

b 13. The tendon begins to develop tears when it is stretched to approximately _____% beyond normal length.
a. 2 to 5
b. 5 to 8
c. 8 to 10
d. 10 to 13

b 14. Strains and sprains that produce moderate discomfort, tenderness, swelling, ecchymosis, detectable joint instability, and/or muscle weakness are categorized as:
a. First-degree injuries
b. Second-degree injuries
c. Third-degree injuries
d. Fourth-degree injuries

a 15. The substance that increases vessel permeability and stimulates nerve endings to cause pain is:
a. Bradykinin
b. Histamine
c. Postaglandins
d. Serotonin

c 16. Longitudinal bone growth occurs at the bone's:
a. Apophyseal plates
b. Cortical plates
c. Epiphyseal plates
d. Periosteal plates

a 17. Remodeling of bone tissue involves osteoblast activity on the _______ side of the fracture.
a. Concave
b. Convex
c. Epiphyseal
d. Tension

d 18. Because the nerve roots on the spinal cord are not protected by connective tissue, they are particularly susceptible to what kind of injury?
a. Compressive
b. Impacted
c. Shearing
d. Tensile

c 19. Random regrowth of a nerve after injury is called a:
a. Hyponeuromesis
b. Hyperneuromesis
c. Neuroma
d. Neurotmesis

a 20. Small diameter, slow transmission nerves carry impulses for what sensation?
a. Pain
b. Proprioception
c. Temperature
d. Touch

MATCHING - Match the correct terms and place the answer in the space provided.

_q_ 1. Afferent nerves
_c_ 2. Anisotropic
_g_ 3. Bending
_m_ 4. Contusion
_t_ 5. Dermatome
_k_ 6. Ecchymosis
_r_ 7. Efferent nerves
_a_ 8. Force
_l_ 9. Hematoma
_n_ 10. Hypoxia
_h_ 11. Ligament
_s_ 12. Nociceptors
_p_ 13. Osteopenia
_o_ 14. Phagocytosis
_e_ 15. Strain
_d_ 16. Stress
_i_ 17. Tendon
_f_ 18. Torque
_j_ 19. Viscoelastic
_b_ 20. Yield point

a. A push or pull acting on a body
b. Maximum load that can be sustained without permanent deformation
c. Having different strengths in response to loads from different directions
d. Distribution of force within a body, or force divided by the surface area over which the force is applied
e. Amount of deformation an object undergoes in response to an applied force
f. A rotary force or the product of a force and its moment arm
g. Loading that produces tension on one side of an object and compression on the other side
h. Tissue that connects bone to bone
i. Tissue that connects muscles to bone
j. Responding to loading over time with changing rates of deformation
k. Superficial tissue discoloration
l. A localized mass of blood and lymph confined within a space or tissue
m. Compression injury involving accumulation of blood and lymph within a muscle
n. Having a reduced concentration of oxygen
o. Process whereby leukocytes ingest dead cells and infectious agents
p. Condition of reduced bone mineral density
q. Nerves carrying sensory input from receptor to the brain
r. Nerves carrying motor stimuli from the brain to the muscles
s. Specialized nerve endings that transmit pain
t. Areas of skin innervated by a single spinal nerve

Chapter 3
Emergency Procedures

c 1. The immediate assessment occurring on the field when a life-threatening injury is present is called:
a. Babinski test
b. CPR
c. Primary survey
d. Secondary survey

d 2. Information provided by the individual regarding their perception of the problem is called a:
a. Primary survey
b. Secondary survey
c. Sign
d. Symptom

c 3. A measurable physical finding regarding the individual's condition is called a:
a. Cyanotic test
b. Level of consciousness
c. Sign
d. Symptom

c 4. The universal distress signal indicates possible:
a. Concussion
b. Heart attack
c. Obstructed airway
d. Shock

a 5. The leading cause of loss of consciousness in a sport activity is due to:
a. Head injuries
b. Heat stroke
c. Metabolic disturbances
d. Spinal injuries

d 6. In medical situations, consciousness is determined through:
a. Level of stupor
b. Tactile stimuli
c. Verbal stimuli
d. Verbal and sensory stimuli

c 7. The best method to control hemorrhage is:
a. Direct pressure
b. Elevation above the heart
c. Direct pressure and elevation above the heart
d. Indirect pressure

d 8. What is hemophilia?
a. Fear of blood
b. Decreased amount of red blood cells
c. Inability of blood to travel to the heart muscle
d. Inability of blood to clot

a 9. Which of the following signs and symptoms is usually not present with internal bleeding in the abdomen?
a. Dull eyes with constricted pupils
b. Nausea and vomiting blood
c. Pale, cold, and clammy skin
d. Rapid, weak pulse

c 10. Metabolic shock results from
a. Excessive blood/fluid loss that leads to inadequate circulation and oxygen supply to all body organs
b. Severe allergic reaction to a foreign protein
c. Severe loss of body fluids due to an untreated illness that alters the biochemical equilibrium
d. Temporary dilation of blood vessels leading to blood draining from the head and pooling in the abdomen

d 11. Which of the following signs and symptoms does not indicate possible shock?
a. Anxiety, restlessness
b. Cold, clammy skin
c. Extreme thirst
d. Rapid, bounding pulse

a 12. Which of the following measures would help prevent the onset of hyperthermia?
a. Acclimate to the environment
b. Eat high carbohydrate foods
c. Ingest a cola soda pop prior to exercising
d. Ingest water only after exercise is completed

a 13. The rate of gastric emptying can be retarded when ingested fluids contain even the smallest amount of:
a. Salt or simple sugar
b. Protein
c. Vitamin A
d. Vitamin K

c 14. In general, water breaks during hot weather should be scheduled every:
a. 10 minutes
b. 15 minutes
c. 20 to 30 minutes
d. every hour

b 15. Fatigue, dizziness, confusion, rapid and shallow respirations, and a rapid, weak pulse are all signs of:
a. Heat cramps
b. Heat exhaustion
c. Heat stroke
d. Prickly heat

b 16. During cold weather, body heat is gained through all of these mechanisms except:
a. Increase in basal metabolism
b. Increased respirations
c. Shivering
d. Thyroxine and epinepherine production

b 17. The most important factor that determines the effectiveness of evaporative heat loss is:
a. Ambient temperature
b. Relative humidity
c. Solar radiant energy
d. Time of day

d 18. Assessing all injured individuals quickly, then returning to the most seriously injured to give them immediate treatment is called:
a. Assessment
b. Primary survey
c. Secondary survey
d. Triage

d 19. If a head or neck injury is suspected, the preferred method to open the airway is the:
a. Finger sweep method
b. Head tilt/chin lift method
c. Heimlich maneuver
d. Jaw thrust method

a 20. Which of the following is not considered to be a vital sign?
a. Pupillary response to light
b. Pulse
c. Respirations
d. Skin temperature

Short Answer: List three conditions that may be indicated when the following abnormal vital signs are present.

Rapid, weak pulse
1.
2.
3.

Slow, bounding pulse
1.
2.
3.

Shallow breathing
1.
2.
3.

Respiratory arrest
1.
2.
3.

Cool, clammy skin
1.
2.
3.

Hot, dry skin
1.
2.
3.

White or ashen skin
1.
2.
3.

Red or flushed skin
1.
2.
3.

ESSAY 1. A football player is lying motionless face up on the turf, but you did not see the injury occur. Explain how you would complete a primary survey of this individual.

ESSAY 2. Using the HOPS format, explain the steps you would perform in completing a secondary survey of the football player. List the questions asked in taking a history, what factors you observe for, how you would palpate for injury, what you are looking for when you palpate, and what special tests you might use to determine the level of consciousness.

ESSAY 3. List and explain the different procedures used to determine a possible fracture.

Chapter 4
Sports Injury Assessment

_a_ 1. As the first person on the scene of a sports related injury, you are expected to:
a. Assess the extent and seriousness of injury
b. Immobilize the joint in the position it was found
c. Notify the parents of a minor child of the injury
d. Summon EMS immediately

_d_ 2. Which of the following is correct?
a. The elbow is proximal to the shoulder
b. The thumb is on the medial side of the hand
c. In anatomical position, the forearms are pronated
d. The knee is proximal to the ankle

_a_ 3. Which of the following terms refers to a structure on both sides of the body or body part?
a. Bilateral
b. Contralateral
c. Ipsilateral
d. Lateral

_a_ 4. Which of the following is **not** a correctly matched pair of terms?
a. Adduction—movement away from the midline of the body
b. Flexion—decreasing an angle
c. Extension—increasing an angle
d. Dorsiflexion—movement of the forefoot toward the shin

_b_ 5. When you are denoting what disease, injury, or syndrome that a person has or is believed to have, you are making a(an):
a. Evaluation
b. Diagnosis
c. Judgment
d. Prognosis

_d_ 6. A noted or subjective change in an individual's body or its functions that indicates an injury or disease is called a(n):
a. Diagnosis
b. Etiology
c. Sign
d. Symptom

_d_ 7. Which of the following should not be done during the history taking of an injury evaluation?
a. Person describes how the injury occurred
b. Person locates the area of pain by pointing to it
c. Person describes past injuries to other body parts
d. Person tries to measure movement of the injured part

_d_ 8. Somatic pain arises from
a. Organs in the abdominal cavity
b. Organs in the thoracic cavity
c. Referred pain sensations when injury to one body part travels up or down the length of a nerve root
d. Skin, ligaments, muscles, bones, and joints

c 9. When asking about the characteristics of symptoms, determine:
a. Limitations in sport, occupational, and ADLs
b. Location, onset, limb position, direction of force
c. Location, onset, severity, frequency, duration
d. Previous injuries, congenital abnormalities, family history

b 10. The visual analysis of overall appearance, symmetry, general motor function, posture, and gait is called:
a. Inspection
b. Observation
c. Proprioceptive input
d. Symptom

b 11. The escape of fluid from the blood vessels into the joint cavity is called:
a. Ecchymosis
b. Effusion
c. Erythema
d. Swelling

c 12. Movement of an affected part by another person or device without effort by the athlete is _________ exercise?
a. Active
b. Assistive
c. Passive
d. Resistive

b 13. Range of motion is measured quantitatively with a:
a. Dynamometer
b. Goniometer
c. Sphygmomanometer
d. Tape measure

a 14. Movements within the joint that cannot be voluntarily performed by the individual are called:
a. Accessory movements
b. Active movements
c. Assistive movements
d. Passive movements

a 15. The position in which two joint surfaces fit precisely together is called the:
a. Closed packed position
b. Firm packed position
c. Loose packed position
d. Packed position

b 16. A muscle that can move through the complete range of motion against gravity, with some resistance is graded as:
a. Fair
b. Good
c. Normal
d. Poor

a 17. An advantage of testing muscle strength throughout the full range of motion is that:
a. A painful arc of motion can be identified
b. It evaluates accessory motions at the joint
c. It occurs in only the loose packed position
d. Overload pressure can be regulated relative to pain

b 18. Which of the following is not a normal joint end feel?
a. Bone to bone
b. Capsular
c. Soft tissue approximation
d. Tissue stretch

d 19. An abnormal sensation characterized by a numbness, tingling, or burning sensation is called:
a. Anesthesia
b. Hypoesthesia
c. Hyperesthesia
d. Paresthesia

a 20. When using SOAP notes, long-term and short-term goals are identified in what section of the documentation?
a. Assessment
b. Objective evaluation
c. Plan
d. Subjective evaluation

MATCHING. Match up the nerve root segment with the action that tests its integrity.

j	1. C3	a. Ankle dorsiflexion
l	2. C4	b. Ankle plantar flexion, eversion
k	3. C5	c. Elbow extension, wrist flexion
d	4. C6	d. Elbow flexion, wrist extension
c	5. C7	e. Finger abduction, adduction
m	6. C8	f. Great toe extension
e	7. T1	g. Hip flexion
g	8. L1-L2	h. Knee extension
h	9. L3	i. Knee flexion
a	10. L4	j. Neck lateral flexion
f	11. L5	k. Shoulder abduction
b	12. S1	l. Shoulder elevation
i	13. S2	m. Thumb extension, ulnar deviation

Essay 1. List and explain the components from the five key areas used to develop a history of an injury.

Essay 2. List at least six characteristics that you could palpate for during bony and soft tissue palpations.

Essay 3. Describe the three normal end feels and briefly explain what each feels like.

CHAPTER 5
THERAPEUTIC EXERCISE AND THERAPEUTIC MODALITIES

_a_ 1. In designing an individualized therapeutic exercise program, the first step is to:
a. Assess the present level of function and dysfunction
b. Develop a treatment plan
c. Establish long-term and short-term goals
d. Formulate a list of patient problems

_c_ 2. Which of the following is not considered to be a long-term goal?
a. Bilateral equal range of motion
b. Maintenance of cardiovascular fitness
c. Control of inflammation
d. Relaxation training

_a_ 3. Which of the following statements is true concerning collagenous scar formation as compared to the original mature injured tissue?
a. It is less efficient and tolerant of tensile forces
b. It is less efficient and tolerant of shearing forces
c. It is more efficient and tolerant of tensile forces
d. It is more efficient and tolerant of shearing forces

_a_ 4. The longer the inflammatory process progresses, what happens to the resulting scar tissue?
a. It will be less dense and weaker in resisting applied stress
b. It will be more dense and stronger in resisting applied stress
c. It will be more dense and weaker to resisting applied stress
d. It will be resistant to applied stress at the same level as the previously injured tissue

_b_ 5. A lower skin temperature can be produced with the application of an:
a. Ice bag applied with a dry elastic wrap
b. Ice bag applied with a wet elastic wrap
c. Ice bag applied over a single layer of clothing
d. Skin temperature remains the same regardless of any layering

_b_ 6. A single application of cold should not extend beyond:
a. 5 to 10 minutes
b. 15 to 30 minutes
c. 30 to 45 minutes
d. 50 to 60 minutes

_d_ 7. In fitting crutches, the hand grips should be placed at a height to allow the elbow to be flexed about:
a. 15 degrees
b. 20 degrees
c. 25 degrees
d. 30 degrees

_a_ 8. Prolonged immobilization can lead to muscles losing their flexibility and assuming a shortened position. This is referred to as a:
a. Contracture
b. Hypomobility
c. Hypermobility
d. Sharpey's fibrosis

_a_ 9. The optimal time for beginning therapeutic exercise is approximately how long after surgery or injury?
a. Immediately after
b. 24 hours later
c. 3 to 4 days later
d. When pain subsides

d 10. A method of promoting or hastening the recovery response of muscles through the use of diagonal or spiral patterns is characteristic of:
a. DeLorme's progressive resistance exercises
b. Hydrotherapeutic exercises
c. Isokinetic exercises
d. Proprioceptive neuromuscular facilitation exercises

c 11. An individual can move into Phase III of the rehabilitation program when what percent of normal passive and active range of motion is achieved?
a. 60% c. 80%
b. 70% d. 90%

c 12. Joint flexibility is a combination of all of the following except:
a. Mobility of soft tissues c. Muscle strength
b. Muscle extensibility d. Normal joint mechanics

b 13. Nonsteroidal anti-inflammatory drugs aid healing by:
a. Decreasing the sensitivity of pain receptors
b. Increasing vasodilation and inhibiting the production of prostaglandins
c. Increasing vasoconstriction and capillary permeability
d. Decreasing muscle extensibility

a 14. General exercises to restore proprioceptive input and improve joint dynamics and coordination are called:
a. Closed chain exercises c. Open chain exercises
b. Isometric exercises d. Plyometric exercises

a 15. Which of the following are physiological effects of cryotherapy?
a. Decreased metabolism, nerve conduction, and pain perception
b. Decreased vasoconstriction, increased nerve conduction velocity, decreased pain perception
c. Increased vasoconstriction and metabolism, decreased pain
d. Increased vasodilation, increased metabolism, decreased capillary permeability

c 16. Which of the following are physiological effects of local heat?
a. Decreased capillary pressure, decreased cell permeability, increased edema
b. Decreased cellular metabolism, capillary permeability, and pain
c. Increased metabolism, analgesia, decreased pain
d. Increased temperature, increased metabolism, increased vasoconstriction

d 17. A technique that temporarily freezes superficial tissues to aid the clinician in reducing the pain-spasm cycle prior to stretching exercises is use of a(n):
a. Contrast baths c. Paraffin bath
b. Ice massage d. Vapocoolant sprays

d 18. A preferred therapeutic massage for areas around joints and other areas where tissue is thin would be:
a. Petrissage c. Effleurage
b. Tapotement d. Friction

a 19. Both microwave and shortwave diathermy generate heat in the body tissues by the action of ________________ waves.
a. Electromagnetic c. Low voltage
b. Ultrasonic d. All of the above

c 20. The introduction of anti-inflammatory drugs through the skin with ultrasound is called:
a. Cavitation c. Phonophoresis
b. Iontophoresis d. TENS

ESSAY 1. List and explain the six steps used to develop a therapeutic exercise program.

ESSAY 2. Explain the four phases of a therapeutic exercise program and briefly state the main goals in each phase.

ESSAY 3. List at least six lower extremity exercises to improve balance and proprioception.

SHORT ANSWER. List at least four indications and four contraindications for the following modalities.

1. Cryotherapy Application
2. Thermotherapy Application
3. Ultrasound
4. Neuromuscular Electrical Stimulation
5. Continuous Passive Mobilization

MATCHING: Match the correct terms and place the answer in the space provided.

h 1. Active inhibition
d 2. Agonist
u 3. Analgesics
b 4. Anesthetics
e 5. Antagonist
f 6. Ballistic stretching
t 7. Cavitation
a 8. Contracture
p 9. Contraindication
n 10. Coordination
q 11. Counterirritant
y 12. Cryokinetics
v 13. Effleurage
c 14. Flexibility
r 15. Hyperemia
o 16. Indication
w 17. Petrissage
m 18. Plyometric training

a. Adhesions in an immobilized muscle leading to a shortened state
b. Drug that prevents pain from being perceived
c. Total motion at a joint
d. Muscle that performs primary movement
e. Muscle that acts in opposition
f. Repetitive bouncing motions to increase flexibility
g. Slow deliberate muscle stretching
h. Individual consciously relaxes a muscle prior to stretching
i. Active contraction of the agonist to cause a reflex relaxation in the antagonist

_i_ 19. Reciprocal inhibition
_g_ 20. Static stretching
_l_ 21. Sticking point
_j_ 22. Strength
_x_ 23. Tapotement
_k_ 24. Valsalva effect
_s_ 25. Wheal

j. Ability to produce force in one maximal effort
k. Holding one's breath against a closed glottis
l. Insufficient strength to move a body segment through a ROM
m. Explosive movements used to develop muscular power
n. Ability to execute smooth, accurate, and controlled movement
o. Condition that could benefit from use of a specific modality
p. Condition that could be harmed by use of a specific modality
q. Substance that irritates superficial sensory nerves
r. Increase of blood into a region once the treatment has ended
s. An elevated, red or white area on the body seen in allergies to mechanical or chemical irritants
t. Gas bubble formation due to nonthermal effects of ultrasound
u. Drug that reduces the response to pain usually by sedation
v. Stroking
w. Kneading
x. Percussion
y. Alternating cold application and exercise

Chapter 6
Protective Equipment

_c_ 1. Injuries concentrated in a smaller area as a result of impact from a low-mass, high-velocity object are called:
a. Axial injuries
b. Diffuse injuries
c. Focal injuries
d. Tensile injuries

_c_ 2. Techniques and equipment used to prevent or protect an injury site are called:
a. Functional devices
b. NOCSAE devices
c. Prophylactic devices
d. Resilience devices

_d_ 3. The organization that defines impact standards for football and baseball/softball helmets is the:
a. American Society for Testing and Material
b. Canadian Standards Association
c. Equipment Certification Council
d. National Operating Committee on Standards for Athletic Equipment

_a_ 4. Materials that absorb more energy from high-impact intensity levels through deformation are called:
a. High-density materials
b. Low-density materials
c. Nonresilient materials
d. Resilient materials

_b_ 5. Ice hockey helmets must meet minimum impact standards and carry the stamp of approval from:
a. American Society for Testing and Material
b. Canadian Standards Association
c. Equipment Certification Council
d. National Operating Committee on Standards for Athletic Equipment

_b_ 6. Face guards on football helmets must be no less than:
a. one bar
b. two bars
c. three bars
d. four bars

_c_ 7. The substance that clear face guards and protective eye wear is made from is:
a. Photocarbonate
b. Plastic
c. Polycarbonate
d. Protective glass

_b_ 8. The most effective type of mouth protection is the:
a. Bimaxillary mouth guard
b. Custom-made mouth guard
c. Stock mouth guard
d. Thermal set mouth guard

_a_ 9. All of the following are advantages of the thermal set mouth guard except:
a. Covers both upper and lower dental arches
b. Has a loop strap
c. Is inexpensive
d. Is readily available

_a_ 10. Posterolateral neck protectors cannot decrease the incidence of cervical injuries due to:
a. Axial loading
b. Hyperextension
c. Lateral flexion
d. Lateral rotation

_a_ 11. In football, the greatest force was placed on which bony process?
a. Acromion process
b. Clavicle
c. Coracoid process
d. Spine of the scapula

_b_ 12. Individuals diagnosed with lateral epicondylitis often wear this type of brace to protect the elbow:
a. Bilateral spring brace
b. Counterforce brace
c. Neoprene sleeve
d. Open-cell pad

_b_ 13. Women with medium sized breasts prefer this type of sport bra:
a. Bras with minor modifications and less elasticity
b. Compressive bras
c. Nonelastic material with wide shoulder straps and bands under the breasts
d. These women need no special support

_a_ 14. Hip spica braces are used to limit:
a. Excessive hip abduction
b. Excessive hip adduction
c. Excessive hip extension
d. Excessive hip flexion

_c_ 15. Knee braces that are designed to protect the medial collateral ligament are called:
a. Derotational
b. Functional
c. Prophylactic
d. Rehabilitative

_d_ 16. Knee braces that provide absolute or relative immobilization are called:
a. Derotational
b. Functional
c. Prophylactic
d. Rehabilitative

_a_ 17. Lace-up ankle braces prevent what motions?
a. All ankle motions
b. Dorsiflexion/inversion
c. Dorsiflexion/plantar flexion
d. Eversion/inversion

_b_ 18. Maximal loss in taping restrictions for both inversion and eversion has been found to occur after how many minutes of exercise?
a. 10 minutes
b. 20 minutes
c. 30 minutes
d. 40 minutes

_c_ 19. To more effectively correct biomechanical malalignment at the foot, these devices should be recommended:
a. Antishock heel lifts
b. Arch supports
c. Rigid orthotics
d. Semirigid orthotics

_b_ 20. To prevent many running injuries, which components of shoe design should you pay particular attention to?
a. Arch support and heel height
b. Heel cushioning and forefoot torsional stiffness
c. Rearfoot width and cushioning
d. Shoe length and width of toe box

ESSAY 1. List five equipment design factors that can reduce the potential for injury.

ESSAY 2. Explain the procedures for fitting a football helmet.

ESSAY 3. Explain the procedures for fitting shoulder pads.

Chapter 7
Foot, Ankle, and Lower Leg

__b__ 1. Which of the following ankle ligaments is not a part of the medial collateral ligament (deltoid ligament)?
a. Anterior tibiotalar ligament
b. Calcaneofibular ligament
c. Tibiocalcaneal ligament
d. Tibionavicular ligament

__a__ 2. The primary support for the medial longitudinal arch is the:
a. Calcaneonavicular ligament
b. Long plantar ligament
c. Short plantar ligament
d. Tibialis posterior muscle tendon

__a__ 3. A highly specialized band of tissue on the plantar surface of the foot that provides support for the longitudinal arch is the:
a. Plantar fascia
b. Plantar ligament
c. Plantar sesamoiditis
d. Plantar vulgaris

__a__ 4. The nerve that innervates the anterior compartment of the lower leg is the:
a. Deep peroneal nerve
b. Saphenous nerve
c. Superficial peroneal nerve
d. Tibial nerve

__b__ 5. Several overuse injuries to the medial aspect of the foot and lower leg have been attributed to:
a. Excessive heel contact
b. Prolonged pronation
c. Prolonged supination
d. Running on the toes

__d__ 6. Hyperextension of the MTP joint of the great toe is called:
a. Claw toe
b. Hammer toe
c. Paronychia
d. Turf toe

__a__ 7. A fungal infection known as tinea pedis causes:
a. Athlete's foot
b. Plantars warts
c. Paronychia
d. Freiberg's disease

__b__ 8. Death of a tissue due to insufficient blood supply is called:
a. Apnea
b. Avascular necrosis
c. Avascular margination
d. Hypoxia

__a__ 9. A minor blow to the fibular head can contuse the:
a. Common peroneal nerve
b. Saphenous nerve
c. Sciatic nerve
d. Tibial nerve

__c__ 10. A direct blow to the anterior shin can typically result in all of the following except:
a. Anterior compartment syndrome
b. Circulatory impairment to the foot
c. Fibular fracture
d. Loss of dorsiflexion

__d__ 11. An inversion ankle sprain results from excessive:
a. Dorsiflexion
b. Plantar flexion
c. Pronation
d. Supination

__a__ 12. As stress is applied to the ankle during plantar flexion and inversion, which ligament is the first to stretch?
a. Anterior talofibular
b. Anterior tibiofibular
c. Calcaneofibular
d. Posterior talofibular

c 13. With excessive dorsiflexion and eversion, the talus is thrust laterally and can:
a. Dislocate the transverse tarsal joint
b. Fracture the medial malleolus
c. Fracture the lateral malleolus
d. Rupture the interosseous membrane

c 14. If this tendon ruptures, collapse of the midfoot and hyperpronation may be visible:
a. Tibialis anterior
b. Flexor hallucis brevis
c. Tibialis posterior
d. Quadratus plantae

c 15. Acute rupture of the Achilles tendon is more commonly seen in individuals between the ages of:
a. 15 to 20
b. 20 to 30
c. 30 to 50
d. over 50

d 16. All of the following signs and symptoms indicate a ruptured Achilles tendon except which one?
a. Excessive passive dorsiflexion
b. Inability to stand on the toes
c. Individual hears or feels a popping sensation
d. Will limp with the foot and leg internally rotated

d 17. All of the following can overload the plantar fascia except which one?
a. Excessive or prolonged pronation
b. Excessive tightness in the Achilles tendon
c. Obesity
d. Over 40 years of age

c 18. Palpable pain just anterior to the Achilles tendon is indicative of irritation to the:
a. Flexor hallucis longus
b. Peroneus longus
c. Retrocalcaneal bursa
d. Achilles tendon

c 19. Excessive or prolonged pronation in running that leads to pain in the distal third of the medial tibial border not associated with a stress fracture is typically:
a. Achilles tenosynovitis
b. Exercise-induced compartment syndrome
c. Medial tibial stress syndrome
d. Plantar fasciitis

c 20. Movement in which direction will isolate the anterior talofibular ligament in an anterior drawer test?
a. Straight anterior movement with slight dorsiflexion
b. Straight anterior movement with slight eversion
c. Straight anterior movement with slight plantar flexion and inversion
d. Straight inversion

MATCHING: Place the letter of the correct definition in the space provided.

s	1. Compartment syndrome	a. Joint joined by fibrous connective tissue
o	2. Deep peroneal nerve	b. Innervates lateral compartment
m	3. Hallux	c. Appears to have an arch when nonweight bearing
n	4. Jone's fracture	d. Combined motions of foot abduction, dorsiflexion, and calcaneal eversion
f	5. Keratolytic agent	e. Flatfoot on weight bearing and nonweight bearing
j	6. Metatarsalgia	f. Substance that softens and dissolves tissue
g	7. Osteochondritis dissecans	g. Inflammation of bone and cartilage that can split into pieces into the joint
h	8. Paronychia	h. Infection in the folds of skin surrounding a toenail
i	9. Plantar fascia	i. Plantar aponeurosis
d	10. Pronation	j. General pain around the metatarsal heads
e	11. Rigid flatfoot	k. Traction-type injury to the calcaneal apophysis
k	12. Sever's disease	l. Sound that indicates possible fracture or tenosynovitis
l	13. Snowball crepitation	m. First or great toe
c	14. Supple flatfoot	n. Transverse stress fracture of the fifth metatarsal
b	15. Superficial peroneal nerve	o. Innervates anterior compartment
p	16. Supination	p. Combined motions of foot adduction, plantar flexion, and calcaneal inversion
a	17. Syndesmosis	q. Achilles tendon rupture
t	18. Tenosynovitis	r. Innervates posterior compartment
q	19. Thompson test	s. Increased intramuscular pressure within a confined space
r	20. Tibial nerve	t. Inflammation of the inner lining of the tendon sheath

ESSAY 1. List and explain the techniques used to determine a possible fracture in the foot and lower leg region. What methods can be used to immobilize a suspected fracture to this area?

ESSAY 2. A football lineman is complaining of extreme pain on the ball of his right foot. Although the pain has been present for almost three weeks, it is particularly bothersome late in the practice when he pushes off the right foot to block an opponent. Using the HOPS format, what specific questions should be asked in taking a history of this injury.

ESSAY 3. An individual has pain in the foot upon arising in the morning, particularly in the proximal medial longitudinal arch. Point tenderness is elicited just over and distal to the medial calcaneal tubercle. Using the HOPS format, evaluate this athlete.

ESSAY 4. List exercises that can increase muscular strength, endurance, and power in the muscles of the foot and lower leg.

ESSAY 5. List the functional tests and criteria you would use to determine when an injured sport participant can return to full participation.

Chapter 8
The Knee

c 1. Because the medial and lateral condyles of the femur differ somewhat in size, shape, and orientation, the tibia rotates laterally on the femur during the last few degrees of extension. This action is known as what?
a. Loose packed position
b. Gliding
c. Screw home mechanism
d. Tibial shift

c 2. The menisci are attached to the superior plateaus of the tibia by what structure?
a. Arcuate ligaments
b. Collateral ligaments
c. Coronary ligaments
d. Cruciate ligaments

c 3. The medial meniscus is attached to the medial collateral ligament and to fibers from the:
a. Anterior cruciate ligament
b. Popliteus
c. Semimembranosus
d. Semitendinosus

d 4. The largest bursa of the body is the:
a. Deep infrapatellar
b. Prepatellar
c. Superficial infrapatellar
d. Suprapatellar

c 5. The strongest ligament at the knee is the:
a. Anterior cruciate
b. Fibular collateral
c. Posterior cruciate
d. Tibial collateral

d 6. A Q-angle greater than ____ degrees can predispose the individual to patellar injuries.
a. 8
b. 11
c. 15
d. 18

b 7. Which nerve innervates the quadriceps?
a. Common peroneal
b. Femoral
c. Obturator
d. Sciatic

b 8. The muscle that unlocks the knee from its closed packed position is the:
a. Gastrocnemius
b. Popliteus
c. Quadriceps
d. Semimembranosus

a 9. A kick or blow to the posterolateral aspect of the knee can contuse which nerve?
a. Common peroneal
b. Obturator
c. Saphenous
d. Tibial

b 10. The most commonly injured bursa by compressive forces at the knee is the:
a. Deep infrapatellar
b. Prepatellar
c. Superficial infrapatellar
d. Suprapatellar

d 11. Anteromedial instability indicates damage to all of the following structures except:
a. Anterior cruciate
b. Medial meniscus
c. Tibial collateral
d. Vastus medialis oblique

d 12. A positive valgus instability test at 30 degrees of flexion indicates damage to what ligament?
a. Anterior cruciate c. Posterior cruciate
b. Fibular collateral d. Tibial collateral

a 13. What ligament is often injured during a cutting maneuver, sudden deceleration, or landing in an off-balance position after a jump?
a. Anterior cruciate c. Posterior cruciate
b. Fibular collateral d. Tibial collateral

d 14. When a force displaces the medial tibia condyle in an anterior external rotated position, what is the primary ligamentous restraint to this motion?
a. Anterior cruciate c. Posterior cruciate
b. Fibular collateral d. Tibial collateral

a 15. The most frequently seen rotatory instability at the knee is ____ instability.
a. Anterolateral c. Posterolateral
b. Anteromedial d. Posteromedial

d 16. The dynamic medial stabilizer of the knee is the:
a. Medial meniscus c. Tibial collateral ligament
b. Medial patellar retinacula d. Vastus medialis oblique

c 17. A condition whereby the lateral retinaculum is tight, or the vastus medialis is weak, leading to lateral excursion and pressure on the lateral facet of the patella is called:
a. Chrondromalacia patellae c. Patellofemoral stress syndrome
b. Iliotibial band friction syndrome d. Subluxed patella

b 18. A traction-type injury to the tibial apophysis where the patellar tendon attaches onto the tibial tuberosity is called:
a. Larsen-Johansson disease c. Patellar tendinitis
b. Osgood-Schlatter disease d. Tibial periostitis

c 19. Posterior swelling may indicate each of the following conditions except:
a. Baker's cyst c. Pes anserinus strain
b. Gastrocnemius strain d. Venous thrombosis

a 20. The patellar tap test is used to indicate:
a. Intra-articular or extra-articular swelling
b. Lateral patellar excursion
c. Patellar fracture
d. Patellar subluxation/dislocation

MATCHING. Place the letter of the correct definition in the space provided.

k 1. Anthralgia
c 2. Anterior cruciate
u 3. Apleys' compression test
h 4. Bucket-handle tear
m 5. Chondral fracture
j 6. Extrasynovial
s 7. Gravity drawer test

a. Fibrocartilaginous discs
b. Structures within the joint capsule joint capsule
c. Prevents anterior displacement of tibia on femur
d. Benign or malignant tumor
e. Pus within a joint cavity

_p_ 8. Hemarthrosis
_b_ 9. Intracapsular
_r_ 10. Lachman's test
_t_ 11. McMurrary's test
_a_ 12. Menisci
_d_ 13. Neoplasm
_v_ 14. Ober's test
_n_ 15. Osteochondral fracture
_o_ 16. Osteochondritis dissecans
_i_ 17. Parrot-beak tear
_w_ 18. Patella compression test
_l_ 19. Patella plica
_q_ 20. Posterior cruciate
_e_ 21. Pyarthrosis
_g_ 22. Valgus
_f_ 23. Varus

f. Force that drives distal body segment medially
g. Force that drives distal body segment laterally
h. Longitudinal meniscal tear
i. Horizontal meniscal tear
j. Structures outside the synovial cavity
k. Severe joint pain
l. Synovial lining fold
m. Fracture involving the articular cartilage
n. Fracture involving the articular cartilage and underlying bone
o. Avascular necrosis of joint cartlage and subchondral bone
p. Blood inside joint capsule
q. Structure that prevents posterior displacement of tibia on the femur
r. Tests anterior cruciate
s. Tests posterior cruciate
t. Tests for meniscus injury in supine position
u. Tests for meniscus injury in prone position
v. Tests for iliotibial band friction syndrome
w. Tests for damage to patellar articular cartilage

ESSAY 1. A field hockey player was struck directly on the patella from a ball. The player immediately dropped to the ground in extreme pain. Using the HOPS format, outline how to assess this injury and determine a possible fracture to the patella. If fractured, how should the limb be immobilized?

ESSAY 2. A basketball player was going in for a layup. As the player decelerated, an audible pop was heard, and the knee collapsed. Using the HOPS format, assess this injury. What possible injury does the player have?

ESSAY 3. A female runner is complaining of pain on the lateral aspect of the knee. The training regimen has significantly increased during the past week. It is particularly bothersome when she runs on the streets facing traffic and in running uphills and downhills. Using the HOPS format, assess this injury. What possible injury does the runner have?

ESSAY 4. A 28-year-old male is complaining of chronic pain deep in the knee on the medial aspect. The pain has been present for several years and comes and goes during various activities. It is particularly bothersome when he plays basketball and flag football. The knee is mildly swollen and slightly warm to the touch. Using the HOPS format, assess this injury. What possible injury might you suspect with these symptoms?

ESSAY 5. A football player has a first-degree anterior cruciate injury. Develop a rehabilitation program to restore any deficits in range of motion, strength, endurance, and power at the knee. What closed chain exercises can be used to improve strength and restore coordination and balance? What cardiovascular fitness activities can be initiated early in the program?

Chapter 9
Thigh, Hip, and Pelvis Injuries

_b_ 1. The weakest component of the femur is the:
a. Femoral head
b. Femoral neck
c. Femoral shaft
d. Supracondylar ridge

_d_ 2. The iliofemoral ligament prevents excessive:
a. Abduction
b. Adduction
c. Hip flexion
d. Hip extension

_c_ 3. The nerve that innervates the hip adductors is the:
a. Common peroneal
b. Femoral
c. Obturator
d. Tibial

_b_ 4. Over development of this muscle(s) can lead to anterior pelvic tilt:
a. Hamstrings
b. Iliopsoas
c. Pectineus
d. Rectus femoris

_d_ 5. In a posterior, superior hip dislocation, which major nerve may be damaged?
a. Femoral
b. Greater saphenous
c. Obturator
d. Sciatic

_a_ 6. A contusion caused by direct compression to an unprotected iliac crest is referred to as a(n):
a. Hip pointer
b. Iliac hematoma
c. Iliac tenosynovitis
d. Myositis ossificans

_b_ 7. A serious condition that may occur after a contusion to the quadriceps muscle group involving abnormal ossification of bone deposition within the muscle tissue is called:
a. Exostosis
b. Myositis ossificans
c. Myochonritis exostosis
d. Osteochondritis

_d_ 8. Runners who cross the feet over their midline during running increase the Q angle and can develop:
a. Gluteus medius strain
b. Iliopsoas bursitis
c. Pes anserinus bursitis
d. Trochanteric bursitis

_d_ 9. In a hip dislocation, when the head of the femur displaces in a posterior superior direction, the leg typically rests in what position?
a. Extended and externally rotated
b. Extended and internally rotated
c. Flexed and externally rotated
d. Flexed and internally rotated

_a_ 10. In a femoral shaft fracture, the thigh appears:
a. Shortened and externally rotated
b. Shortened and internally rotated
c. Is the same length, but externally rotated
d. Is the same length, but internally rotated

_d_ 11. The tibial nerve innervates all of the hamstrings except the:
a. Long head of the biceps femoris
b. Semimembranosus
c. Semitendinosus
d. Short head of the biceps femoris

b 12. An individual who complains of sharp groin pain and weakness when running sideways, but not straight-ahead may have a strain to the:
a. Abductor muscles
b. Adductor muscles
c. Iliopsoas complex
d. Rectus femoris

c 13. A strain to what muscle(s) would cause palpable pain in the midbuttock region that worsens at night and may produce weakness or numbness extending down the back of the leg?
a. Adductor magnus
b. Biceps femoris
c. Piriformis
d. Semimembranosus

b 14. Avascular necrosis of the proximal femoral epiphysis is called:
a. Larsen-Johansson disease
b. Legg-Calvé Perthes disease
c. Osgood-Schlatter disease
d. Osteochondritis dissecans

c 15. An acute inflammation of a vein is called a(an):
a. Arteriosclerosis
b. Phlebothrombosis
c. Thrombophlebitis
d. Venous cavitation

d 16. A blood clot that travels through the circulatory system to lodge in a blood vessel in the lungs is called a(n):
a. Arteriosclerosis
b. Arterioplasty
c. Pulmonary arteritis
d. Pulmonary embolism

c 17. An avulsion fracture at the anterior superior iliac spine may involve which muscle?
a. Pectineus
b. Rectus femoris
c. Sartorius
d. Vastus intermedius

d 18. All of the following are frequent complaints with a stress fracture to the pubis or femoral neck except:
a. Inguinal pain
b. Night pain
c. Pain on hip rotation
d. Pain while using the flutter kick when swimming

b 19. It is not unusual that severe bleeding after a femoral fracture can lead to:
a. Analphylactic shock
b. Hypovolemic shock
c. Metabolic shock
d. Septic shock

c 20. The positive Faber's (Patrick's) test may indicate all of the following except:
a. Hip joint contracture
b. Iliopsoas spasm
c. Iliotibial band syndrome
d. Tight piriformis muscle

MATCHING. Match up these tests with the appropriate myotome or special test.

f	1.	Ankle dorsiflexion	a. Rectus femoris contracture
b	2.	Gapping test	b. Anterior sacroiliac ligament sprain
h	3.	Hip extension	c. Posterior sacroiliac ligament sprain
d	4.	Hip flexion	d. Myotome for L_1-L_2
l	5.	Homan's sign	e. Myotome for L_3
a	6.	Kendall's test	f. Myotome for L_4
e	7.	Knee extension	g. Myotome for L_5
i	8.	Knee flexion	h. Myotome for S_1
k	9.	Lasègue's test	i. Myotome for S_2
c	10.	Squish test	j. Flexion contractures
j	11.	Thomas' test	k. Tight hamstrings or stretching of the dura mater
g	12.	Toe extension	l. Deep venous thrombosis

ESSAY 1. Describe several exercises that can be used to prevent injury at the thigh, hip, and pelvis region.

ESSAY 2. A baseball player was struck in the thigh by a line drive. Explain on-the-field management of this injury and what signs and symptoms would indicate that this injury is not a simple contusion.

ESSAY 3. A runner is complaining of chronic pain on the posterior distal thigh. It is particularly painful when running up hills and during overstriding and wind sprints. What primary muscle group has been strained? Using the HOPS format, assess this injury and develop a treatment plan that includes flexibility exercises for the appropriate muscle groups.

ESSAY 4. An adolescent boy is limping and complaining of vague groin pain that has progressively increased in the last three weeks. Examination reveals limited hip abduction, extension, and external rotation. Using the HOPS format, complete this injury assessment. What condition might you be dealing with? What is your immediate course of action?

ESSAY 5. Describe the techniques that can be used to determine a possible stress fracture in the hip region and a femoral fracture.

Chapter 10
Shoulder Injuries

_a_ 1. The ligament that resists independent upward movement of the distal clavicle is the:
a. Acromioclavicular
b. Coracoclavicular
c. Costoclavicular
d. Sternoclavicular

_c_ 2. Which of the following muscles is not a part of the rotator cuff?
a. Subscapularis
b. Supraspinatus
c. Teres major
d. Teres minor

_a_ 3. The main function of the rotator cuff muscles is to:
a. Hold the head of the humerus in the glenoid fossa
b. Perform abduction and external rotation
c. Perform abduction and internal rotation d. Facilitate scapulothoracic motions

_b_ 4. The most commonly injured bursa in the shoulder is the:
a. Biceps bursa
b. Subacromial bursa
c. Subcoracoid bursa
d. Subscapularis bursa

_b_ 5. The brachial plexus is made from what levels of spinal nerves?
a. C_4-T_2
b. C_5-T_1
c. C_5-T_2
d. C_6-T_1

_c_ 6. Which muscle(s) plays a major role in positioning the scapula to facilitate the throwing motion?
a. Latissimus dorsi
b. Levator scapulae
c. Rhomboideus
d. Trapezius

_c_ 7. Which muscle does not serve an important function in preventing impingement of the supraspinatus and subacromial bursa during the throwing motion?
a. Infraspinatus
b. Subscapularis
c. Teres major
d. Teres minor

_b_ 8. Nearly all injuries at the SC joint result from:
a. Bending
b. Compression
c. Shear
d. Tension

_d_ 9. In a moderate AC joint sprain, what motion will cause increased pain and a snapping sound at the joint?
a. Glenohumeral flexion
b. Glenohumeral rotation
c. Horizontal abduction
d. Horizontal adduction

_c_ 10. In a glenohumeral dislocation, the glenoid labrum can be damaged or avulsed from the anterior lip of the glenoid fossa, leading to what type of injury?
a. Anterior deformity
b. Anterior stress lesion
c. Bankart lesion
d. Impingement lesion

_a_ 11. What nerve can be damaged in an anterior glenohumeral dislocation?
a. Axillary nerve
b. Median nerve
c. Musculocutaneous nerve
d. Radial nerve

_a_ 12. In a first time glenohumeral dislocation, the injured arm is usually held in what position?
a. Slightly abducted and externally rotated
b. Slightly abducted and internally rotated
c. Slighted extended and internally rotated
d. Slighted extended in neutral position

_c_ 13. In a rotator cuff strain, pain increases when the arm moves actively between what degrees of abduction?
a. 00 to 30°
b. 40 to 70°
c. 70 to 120°
d. 120 to 180°

_b_ 14. Which of the following structures is usually not injured with an impinge ment syndrome?
a. Long head of biceps brachii
b. Short head of biceps brachii
c. Subacromial bursa
d. Supraspinatus

_c_ 15. Nearly 80% of all clavicular fractures occur where?
a. At the acromion process
b. Medial one third
c. Middle one third
d. Distal one third

_b_ 16. Intra-articular swelling at the glenohumeral joint would prevent the individual from placing the arm in what position?
a. Fully abducted
b. Fully adducted
c. Fully extended
d. Fully flexed

_c_ 17. A more effective method of testing the integrity of the biceps brachii tendon is the:
a. Biceps brachii reflex test
b. Impingement test
c. Speed's test
d. Yergason's test

_d_ 18. Damage to the long thoracic nerve will be evident in:
a. Weakness in scapular elevation
b. Weakness in biceps brachii reflex test
c. Weakness in glenohumeral abduction
d. Winging of the scapula

_d_ 19. A condition whereby nerves and/or vessels become compressed in the root of the neck or axilla, leading to numbness in the arm is called:
a. Dead arm syndrome
b. Impingement syndrome
c. Little league shoulder
d. Thoracic outlet syndrome

_b_ 20. Circumduction and pendulum swings are examples of range of motion exercises collectively known as:
a. Closed chain exercises
b. Codman's exercises
c. Theraband exercises
d. T-bar exercises

MATCHING: Match the correct terms and place the answer in the space provided.

_c_	1. Anterior shoulder dislocation	a. Soft tissue lip around periphery of glenoid
_n_	2. Apley's scratch test	b. Prevents superior excursion of humeral head
_m_	3. Centinela test	c. Apprehension test
_o_	4. Dead arm syndrome	d. Bicipital tendinitis
_h_	5. Elbow extension	e. C4 myotome
_g_	6. Elbow flexion	f. C5 myotome
_j_	7. Finger abduction/adduction	g. C6 myotome
_f_	8. Glenohumeral abduction	h. C7 myotome
_a_	9. Glenoid labrum	i. C8 myotome
_t_	10. Halstead maneuver	j. T1 myotome
_b_	11. Infraspinatus	k. Neurovascular compression
_s_	12. Little league shoulder	l. Impingement syndrome
_q_	13. Scapular adduction	m. Supraspinatus injury
_e_	14. Scapular elevation	n. Active range of motion
_r_	15. Serratus anterior weakness	o. Recurrent anterior shoulder dislocations
_d_	16. Speed's test	p. Drop arm test
_p_	17. Supraspinatus	q. Rhomboideus
_l_	18. Swimmer's shoulder	r. Winging of the scapula
_k_	19. Thoracic outlet syndrome	s. Fracture to proximal humeral growth plate
_i_	20. Thumb extension	t. Technique involving traction on arm with head rotated to opposite side and hyperex tended while taking a pulse

ESSAY 1. Describe how to measure gross range of motion at the glenohumeral joint.

ESSAY 2. Describe how to assess neurologic function at the shoulder using reflex, myotome, and dermatome testing.

ESSAY 3. A swimmer is complaining of anterior shoulder pain that is particularly bothersome during the butterfly stroke. Pain is centered on the anterior lip of the acromion process, and it hurts to do active horizontal adduction across the chest. Using the HOPS format, assess this injury. What possible condition is present?

ESSAY 4. A weight lifter is complaining of a rapid onset of fatigue and an aching pain and numbness in the right side of the neck that extends across the shoulder down the medial arm to the ulnar aspect of the right hand. The symptoms occur after one set of overhead lifting. Using the HOPS format, assess this injury. What possible condition is present?

ESSAY 5. List and explain several closed chain exercises that can be used at the shoulder region.

Chapter 11
Upper Arm, Elbow, and Forearm Injuries

_b_ 1. The angle between the longitudinal axes of the humerus and the ulna when the arm is in anatomical position is known as the:
a. Axial angle
b. Carrying angle
c. Humeroulnar angle
d. Supinated angle

_a_ 2. The ligament that stabilizes and encircles the head of the radius is the:
a. Annular ligament
b. Radial collateral
c. Ulnar collateral
d. Quadrate ligament

_c_ 3. What nerve innervates the main elbow flexors?
a. Axillary
b. Median
c. Musculocutaneous
d. Radial

_c_ 4. What nerve innervates the main elbow extensors?
a. Median
b. Musculocutaneous
c. Radial
d. Ulnar

_d_ 5. Which of the following is not a primary elbow flexor?
a. Brachialis
b. Brachioradialis
c. Biceps brachii
d. Coracobrachialis

_d_ 6. Football linemen who consistently block with their arms may develop an ectopic formation directly on the distal humerus commonly called:
a. Blocker's contusion
b. Blocker's myositis
c. Myositis ossificans
d. Tackler's exostosis

_a_ 7. After a hyperextension injury, palpable anterior joint pain, particularly on the anteromedial side, is more commonly attributed to acute:
a. Anterior capsulitis
b. Arterial impairment
c. Collateral ligament damage
d. Ulnar nerve compression

_d_ 8. Most elbow dislocations occur from axial loading when falling on an outstretched hand, which results in the ulna and radius dislocating:
a. Anteriorly
b. Laterally
c. Medially
d. Posteriorly

_d_ 9. With an elbow dislocation, the arm is frequently held in what position?
a. Extended with the forearm supinated
b. Extended with the forearm appearing shortened
c. Slightly flexed with the forearm pronated
d. Slightly flexed with the forearm appearing shortened

_d_ 10. Recurrent elbow dislocations are usually due to instability that results from disruption of the:
a. Annular ligament
b. Articular cartilage
c. Radial collateral ligament
d. Ulnar collateral ligament

_d_ 11. If an athlete complains of burning, tingling or paresthesia to the fourth and fifth fingers, what structure may be damaged?
a. Flexor digiti minimi
b. Interosseus muscles
c. Median nerve
d. Ulnar nerve

_c_ 12. A rupture of the biceps tendon is usually associated with what mechanism?
a. Elbow hyperextension
b. Elbow hyperflexion
c. Forceful shoulder flexion against excessive resistance
d. Forceful shoulder extension against excessive resistance

_d_ 13. Medial epicondylitis is often caused by what mechanism?
a. Bending
b. Compression
c. Shear
d. Tension

_d_ 14. With moderate medial epicondylitis, throwing or overhead motions should be avoided for up to how many weeks post injury?
a. Can begin immediately
b. 1 to 2 weeks
c. 3 to 4 weeks
d. 6 to 12 weeks

_a_ 15. All of the following mechanisms can lead to common extensor tendinitis except:
a. Eccentric loading of the flexor muscles
b. Excessive use of a curveball
c. Impact forces
d. Use of power grips

_d_ 16. Compression due to hypertrophy of this muscle can impinge the median nerve, leading to weakness in the finger flexors?
a. Brachialis
b. Flexor carpi radialis
c. Flexor carpi ulnaris
d. Pronator teres

_d_ 17. A complication from a forearm fracture that can lead to ischemic necrosis of the forearm muscles is called:
a. Forearm splints
b. Little league elbow
c. Nightstick fracture
d. Volkmann's contracture

_c_ 18. A valgus stress applied at 15 to 20° of elbow flexion stresses what structure?
a. Elbow flexors
b. Radial collateral ligament
c. Ulnar collateral ligament
d. Ulnar nerve

_b_ 19. If resisted wrist extension is applied to an athlete's hand with the forearm pronated and elbow flexed at 45°, what test is being performed?
a. Capsular pain test
b. Common extensor tendinitis test
c. Thomas test
d. Tinel's test

_c__ 20. The adolescent athlete who complains of sudden pain and locking of the elbow joint should be suspected of having:
a. Epicondylitis
b. Olecranon bursitis
c. Osteochondritis dissecans
d. Supracondylar fracture of humerus

MATCHING: Match the correct terms and place the answer in the space provided.

_i_ 1. Biceps brachii
_c_ 2. Brachialis
_j_ 3. Brachioradialis
_b_ 4. Carrying angle
_p_ 5. Coffee cup test
_q_ 6. Cubital valgus
_r_ 7. Cubital varus
_d_ 8. Ectopic bone
_a_ 9. Epicondylitis
_g_ 10. Fibrositis
_o_ 11. Forearm splints
_l_ 12. Little league elbow
_h_ 13. Malaise
_f_ 14. Periostitis
_l_ 15. Pronator syndrome
_e_ 16. Tackler's exostosis
_m_ 17. Tinel's sign
_n_ 18. Wrist drop

a. Inflammation of the soft tissues on the epicondyles at the distal humerus
b. Angle between humerus and ulna in anatomical position
c. Primary elbow flexor
d. Bone ossification in an abnormal place
e. Bone formation on anterior or lateral humerus
f. Inflammation of outer covering of a bone
g. Inflammation of fibrous tissue
h. General discomfort
i. C5 reflex
j. C6 reflex
k. Tension stress injury of the medial epicondyle
l. Median nerve damaged
m. Ulnar nerve damaged
n. Radial nerve damaged
o. Chronic strain of forearm muscles
p. Lateral epicondylitis
q. Carrying angle > 20°
r. Carrying angle < 10°

ESSAY 1. A tennis player has an elbow extensor strain. Outline the immediate treatment and rehabilitation program for this individual. Give specific exercises that should be included in the program.

ESSAY 2. Describe how to assess neural damage and circulatory impairment in the arm after a posterior elbow dislocation.

ESSAY 3. Describe how to determine a possible fracture at the elbow and forearm.

ESSAY 4. A football player is complaining of pain in the anterior distal arm just proximal to the elbow joint. Palpation reveals a hardened mass of soft tissue that is very sore and tender. What specific questions should be asked to gather a history of this injury?

ESSAY 5. A baseball pitcher is complaining of diffuse elbow pain during the throwing motion, particularly on the medial aspect of the joint line that has been getting progressively worse. Numbness and a tingling sensation occasionally occur down the medial aspect of the forearm into the fourth and fifth fingers. Using the HOPS format, assess this injury. What structures may be damaged with this injury?

Chapter 12
Wrist and Hand Injuries

_a_ 1. Flexion of the DIP and PIP joints tests damage to which nerve:
a. Median c. Ulnar
b. Radial d. Volar

_b_ 2. Extension of the thumb and fingers tests damage to which nerve:
a. Median c. Ulnar
b. Radial d. Volar

_b_ 3. Specialized connective tissue that forms protective passageways through which tendons, nerves, and blood vessels pass is called:
a. Carpal tunnels c. Tendinous tunnels
b. Retinacula d. Tunneloses

_a_ 4. All of the following muscles are wrist flexors except:
a. Brachioradialis c. Flexor carpi ulnaris
b. Flexor carpi radialis d. Palmaris longus

_d_ 5. A sprain of the ulnar collateral ligament of the MP joint of the thumb caused by forceful abduction of the thumb while the thumb is extended is called:
a. Baseball thumb c. Bowler's thumb
b. Boutonniere thumb d. Gamekeeper's thumb

_a_ 6. All of the following mechanisms can lead to an interphalangeal collateral ligament sprain except:
a. Compression c. Excessive varus force
b. Excessive valgus force d. Hyperextension

_b_ 7. To ensure the most complete healing of a dislocated PIP joint, the finger should be splinted in about 30° of flexion with active motion starting after:
a. 4 to 9 days c. 15 to 36 days
b. 10 to 14 days d. 37 to 60 days

_b_ 8. The bone most commonly dislocated during axial loading on an extended wrist is the:
a. Capitate c. Scaphoid
b. Lunate d. Triquetrium

_c_ 9. A fixed flexion deformity at the PIP joint of a finger due to inadequate care is called a:
a. Bowler's finger c. Coach's finger
b. Boxer's finger d. Volar's finger

_c_ 10. An inability to flex the distal phalanx due to a rupture of the tendon is called:
a. Boutonniere deformity c. Jersey finger
b. Bowler's finger d. Mallet finger

_a_ 11. A deformity caused by a rupture of the extensor tendon of the middle phalanx is called:
a. Boutonniere deformity
b. Bowler's finger
c. Handlebar's palsy
d. Mallet finger

_b_ 12. Stenosing tenosynovitis of the first tunnel of the wrist through which the extensor pollicis brevis and abductor pollicis longus move is characteristic of:
a. Bowler's thumb
b. de Quervain's disease
c. Forearm splints
d. Volkmann's contractures

_b_ 13. Tapping sign over the transverse carpal ligament tests for:
a. Arterial impingement
b. Carpal tunnel syndrome
c. Ganglions
d. Tenosynovitis of the flexor tendons

_d_ 14. A softball catcher is complaining of swelling over the hypothenar mass and numbness in the little finger. What structure may be damaged?
a. Carpal tunnel
b. Median nerve
c. Radial nerve
d. Ulnar nerve

_b_ 15. A wrist fracture where the radius and ulna are forced dorsally is called a:
a. Bowler's fracture
b. Colles' fracture
c. de Quervain's fracture
d. Smith fracture

_d_ 16. Possible complications of a forearm fracture are muscle spasm, swelling, or arterial damage that inhibits blood circulation to the wrist and hand. This complication is called:
a. Colles' fracture
b. Compartment syndrome
c. Smith's fracture
d. Volkmann's contracture

_c_ 17. Severe point tenderness in the anatomical "snuffbox" may indicate a fracture of which bone?
a. Hamate
b. Lunate
c. Scaphoid
d. Trapezoid

_a_ 18. An articular fracture-dislocation to the proximal end of the first metacarpal is called a(n):
a. Bennett's fracture
b. Bowler's fracture
c. Galeazzi fracture
d. Monteggia fracture

_c_ 19. Which of the following tests may be used to determine if the median or ulnar nerves are compressed?
a. Allen's test
b. de Quervain's test
c. Phalen's test
d. Tinel's sign

_b_ 20. A test used to determine possible de Quervain's tenosynovitis is the:
a. Carpal tunnel compression test
b. Finkelstein test
c. Froment's test
d. Phalen's test

MATCHING: Match the correct terms and place the answer in the space provided.

_m_ 1. Aseptic necrosis
_l_ 2. Bowler's thumb
_k_ 3. Cyclist's palsy
_b_ 4. Dorsal
_j_ 5. Felon
_g_ 6. Ganglion
_n_ 7. Hypothenar
_c_ 8. Jersey finger
_d_ 9. Mallet finger
_i_ 10. Paronychia
_f_ 11. Stenosing
_h_ 12. Subungual hematoma
_o_ 13. Thenar
_e_ 14. Trigger finger
_a_ 15. Volar

a. Referring to palm of hand
b. Referring to back of hand
c. Rupture of flexor tendon from distal phalanx
d. Rupture of extensor tendon from distal phalanx
e. Snapping flexor tendons
f. Narrowing of an opening
g. Benign tumor mass
h. Blood under fingernail
i. Infection along nail fold
j. Abscess within fat pad
k. Results in paresthesia in the ulnar nerve pattern
l. Compression of digital nerve on the medial thumb
m. Death or decay of tissue due to poor blood supply
n. Little finger muscle mass
o. Thumb muscle mass

_j_ 1. Bennett's fracture
_f_ 2. Boutonniere deformity
_i_ 3. Boxer's fracture
_b_ 4. Coach's finger
_e_ 5. Colles' fracture
_k_ 6. Finkelstein test
_o_ 7. Froment's sign
_d_ 8. Galeazzi fracture
_h_ 9. Gamekeeper's thumb
_a_ 10. Monteggia fracture
_c_ 11. Osteomyelitis
_l_ 12. Phalen's test
_n_ 13. Pinch grip test
_g_ 14. Smith fracture
_m_ 15. Tinel's sign

a. Ulnar fracture with radial head dislocation
b. Fixed flexion deformity due to dislocation at PIP
c. Infection of the bone
d. Radial fracture with ulna dislocation at distal end
e. Radius and ulna dorsally angulated fracture
f. Rupture of central slip of extensor tendon at middle phalanx
g. Radius and ulna with volar angulated fracture
h. Rupture of volar ligament at the MP joint of thumb
i. Fracture of 5th metacarpal with rotation of the head over the neck
j. Fracture-dislocation of proximal thumb joint (CM)
k. De Quervain's tenosynovitis

l. Median and ulnar nerve compression
m. Median nerve compression in carpal tunnel
n. Anterior interosseus nerve entrapment
o. Ulnar nerve paralysis

ESSAY 1. Describe what precautions can be taken to prevent injury to the wrist and hand.

ESSAY 2. Describe what factors should be observed and inspected for when assessing a hand or finger injury.

ESSAY 3. Describe how to determine a possible fracture at the wrist and hand.

ESSAY 4. An individual is complaining that numbness and tingling in the wrist wakes him/her in the middle of the night, and the individual has to shake the hand to get the feeling back. It hurts to flex the fingers, and the condition is progressively getting worse. Using the HOPS format assess this injury and identify what possible condition this individual has.

ESSAY 5. Describe a total rehabilitation program for the wrist and hand, giving specific exercises used in each of the phases.

Chapter 13
Head and Facial Injuries

c 1. The outermost meninges that is a dense, fibrous, sheath hat encloses the brain and cord is the:
a. Arachnoid
b. Cerebral cortex
c. Dura mater
d. Pia mater

a 2. Which of the following statements is not related to the conjunctiva of the eye?
a. Continually releases tears to cleanse the eye and keep it moist
b. Lines the eyelids and external surface of the eye
c. Reduces friction between the eyelids and external surface of the eye
d. Secretes mucus to lubricate the external eye

d 3. Which of the following cranial nerves is responsible for motor supply to the jaw muscles and sensation to the facial region?
a. Facial
b. Hypoglossal
c. Olfactory
d. Trigeminal

c 4. What artery is commonly injured in a head injury and, if torn, can lead to an epidural hematoma?
a. Facial artery
b. Vertebral artery
c. Middle meningeal artery
d. Anterior cerebral artery

c 5. Which of the following injuries is responsible for over two-thirds of all head injury deaths?
a. Contrecoup injuries
b. Diffuse injuries
c. Focal injuries
d. Mechanical injuries

b 6. A danger with open fractures to the skull is the greater risk of a bacterial infection that can lead to:
a. Fovea chylamadia
b. Meningitis
c. Tinea capitis
d. Verrucae capitis

a 7. Raccoon eyes are characteristic of what injury?
a. Fracture of the anterior cranial fossa and sinuses
b. Fracture of the ethmoid bone.
c. Fracture of the floor of the occiput
d. Fracture of the nasal region

b 8. "Targeting" or the "halo test" is used to determine the presence of:
a. Blood in the ear
b. CSF in the ear
c. Blood in the nasal septum
d. Inner ear infection

c 9. Treatment for an epidural hematoma is:
a. After completing special tests, return them to play
b. Ice on the injured area and reevaluate in 20 minutes
c. Immediate surgery to decompress the skull
d. Rest and observation

a 10. When an individual has slight mental confusion, dizziness, minimal unsteadiness, and a brief loss of judgment, they have what grade of concussion?
a. Grade I
b. Grade II
c. Grade III
d. Grade IV

a 11. After the first episode of a grade II concussion, the individual may return to play when:
a. Asymptomatic for 1 week
b. May return to play that day
c. May return to play the next day
d. Never; terminate the season

d 12. Which of the following signs and symptoms are characteristic of a Grade III concussion?
a. Decortication
b. Postconcussion syndrome
c. Post-traumatic memory loss
d. Retrograde amnesia

b 13. Once at the site of an unconscious athlete, you should first:
a. Call a physician
b. Look for the possibility of impaired breathing
c. Remove any protective equipment such as a helmet
d. Roll the athlete face up and start CPR

a 14. Which of the following responses are not a part of the Glasgow Coma Scale?
a. Best cutaneous sensation response
b. Best motor response
c. Best verbal response
d. Opening the eyes

b 15. An individual who develops post-traumatic amnesia and postconcussion syndrome is graded at what level of concussion?
a. Grade I
b. Grade II
c. Grade III
d. Grade IV

b 16. A test used to determine the degree of balance difficulties in a grade II concussion is the:
a. Babinski test
b. Romberg test
c. Thompson test
d. Tinel test

b 17. After impact, the brain continues to accelerate and rotate causing tearing of the veins away from the actual injury site, which can lead to a ___ injury.
a. Cerebral
b. Contrecoup
c. Direct
d. Whiplash

a 18. A common sign of a facial fracture to the maxilla or mandible, or a temporomandibular dislocation is:
a. Malocclusion
b. Nosebleed
c. Raccoon eyes
d. Sunken eye

a 19. Which of the following should not be done when managing a bleeding nose?
a. Tilt the head back to decrease bleeding
b. Lie on the same side as the bleeding septum
c. Place a cold compress over the nasal junction
d. Apply finger pressure to the affected nostril for 5 minutes

d 20. Localized infections of the middle ear secondary to upper respiratory infections is called:
a. Otitis externa
b. Otitis intermedius
c. Otitis interna
d. Otitis media

MATCHING: Place the letter of the correct response in the space provided.

f	1. Battle's sign	a. Injuries away from the actual injury site
h	2. Comminuted fractures	b. Localized cerebral damage
u	3. Conjunctivitis	c. Widespread cerebral damage
a	4. Contrecoup	d. Inflammation of the meninges of the brain
i	5. Depressed fractures	e. Discoloration around eyes
c	6. Diffuse injuries	f. Discoloration behind ears
x	7. Diplopia	g. Fracture in a line
j	8. Dyspnea	h. Fracture in multiple pieces
p	9. Epistaxis	i. Fracture with pieces driven internally
b	10. Focal injuries	j. Shortness of breath
w	11. Hyphema	k. Balance disturbance
g	12. Linear fractures	l. Sensitivity to light
o	13. Malocclusion	m. Ringing in the ear
d	14. Meningitis	n. Abnormal eye movement
y	15. Myopia	o. Inability to bring the teeth together
n	16. Nystagmus	p. Nosebleed
s	17. Otitis externa	q. Middle ear infection
q	18. Otitis media	r. Fluid buildup behind ear drum
t	19. Periorbital ecchymosis	s. Infection of the lining of the auditory canal
l	20. Photophobia	t. Black eye
e	21. Raccoon eyes	u. Pinkeye
r	22. Serous otitis	v. Infection of sebaceous gland of an eyelash
v	23. Sty	w. Hemorrhage into the anterior chamber of the eye
m	24. Tinnitus	
k	25. Vertigo	x. Double vision
		y. Near sightedness

ESSAY 1. A basketball player took an elbow to the nasal area, and the nose is now bleeding. Using the HOPS format, assess this injury to determine a possible nasal fracture and describe the different methods used to stop nasal bleeding.

ESSAY 2. A softball player slid into second base and collided with the shortstop. The player's glove (with the ball in it) grazed the player's face. Time-out has been called on the field because your team's player has cupped both of her hands over her eyes and appears to be in pain. Using the HOPS format, assess this injury and describe what immediate treatment is necessary.

ESSAY 3. Identify the signs and symptoms of a possible skull fracture. What steps should be taken to manage the injury?

ESSAY 4. During a soccer game, two players collide trying to head the ball, impacting their heads together. Both go down, but the opponent shakes his head and gets up to continue play. Your team's player remains motionless on the ground facedown. You are called onto the field to care for the athlete. Using the Glasgow Coma Scale, how will you assess the level of consciousness?

ESSAY 5. List at least four signs and symptoms that would indicate that immediate medical referral is necessary in each of the following facial regions.

a. Nasal region
b. Oral and dental region
c. Ear region
d. Eye region

Chapter 14
Injuries to the Spine

c 1. The functional unit of the spine is called the:
a. Intervertebral disc
b. Ligamentum nuchae
c. Motion segment
d. Vertebrae

b 2. The vertebrae that consists of a bony ring with large, flat, superior articular facets on which the skull rests is the:
a. Annulus fibrosis
b. Atlas
c. Axis
d. Dens

b 3. The ligament that connects the pedicles of the adjacent vertebrae is the:
a. Interspinous ligament
b. Ligamentum flavum
c. Posterior longitudinal ligament
d. Supraspinous ligament

c 4. Lateral rotational curvature of the spine is called:
a. Kyphosis
b. Lordosis
c. Scoliosis
d. Spondylolysis

b 5. Actions involving stimulation of a motor neuron by a sensory neuron in the spinal cord without involvement of the brain are called:
a. Cauda equina
b. Reflexes
c. Segmental nerves
d. Spinal nerves

a 6. When the body is in an upright position, the line of gravity passes where in relation to the spinal column?
a. Anterior to the spinal column
b. Posterior to the spinal column
c. Through the middle of the lumbar vertebrae
d. Through the middle of the thoracic vertebrae

a 7. The region of the vertebrae most susceptible to stress fracture is the:
a. Pars interarticularis
b. The body
c. The pedicle
d. Vertebral arch

c 8. A bilateral separation in the pars interarticularis that leads to anterior displacement of a vertebra is:
a. Lordosis
b. Spina bifida
c. Spondylolisthesis
d. Spondylolysis

d 9. A loss of cerebrospinal fluid around the spinal cord due to deformation of the spinal cord or a narrowing of the neural canal is called:
a. Spina bifida
b. Scheuermann's disease
c. Spinal occlusion
d. Spinal stenosis

d 10. Bilateral sensory changes including burning pain, tingling, or total loss of sensation is referred to as:
a. Burner
b. Cervical dislocation
c. Cervical fracture
d. Neuropraxia

b 11. If a unilateral cervical dislocation is present, the neck will be visibly tilted in what direction?
a. Away from the dislocated side
b. Toward the dislocated side
c. Toward extension of the neck
d. Toward flexion of the neck

d 12. Which of the following signs or symptoms would not indicate a cervical spinal injury?
a. Muscular weakness in extremities
b. Absent or weak reflexes
c. Sensory changes in the upper clavicular area
d. Positive Babinski's test

a 13. With a brachial plexus injury, the injury usually affects what nerve roots of the plexus?
a. C_5-C_6
b. C_6-C_7
c. C_7-C_8
d. C_8-T_1

c 14. A condition of reduced bone mineralization, more commonly seen in women, in the lumbar region is called:
a. Anemia
b. Osteochondritis dessicans
c. Osteopoenia
d. Scheuermann's disease

a 15. When disc nuclear material moves into the spinal canal and impinges adjacent nerve roots, it is called a(n):
a. Extruded disc
b. Herniated disc
c. Prolapsed disc
d. Sequestrated disc

b 16. If an individual has a diminished quadriceps reflex and weak ankle dorsiflexion, what nerve root is injured?
a. L3
b. L4
c. L5
d. S1

b 17. In sciatica with sensory and reflex changes, muscle weakness, and normal bowel and bladder function present, the person may return to sport participation in:
a. 6 to 12 weeks
b. 12 to 24 weeks
c. After surgical decompression and rehabilitation
d. They probably will never return to sport activity

c 18. The top of the iliac crest is the landmark for which vertebrae?
a. T12
b. L2
c. L4
d. S1

a 19. Hip flexion tests which nerve root myotome segment?
a. L1-L2
b. L3
c. L5
d. S1

c 20. Ipsilateral pain during the first 70 degrees of a straight leg raising test indicates a possible:
a. Herniated disc
b. Irritation of the sacroiliac joint
c. Sciatica
d. Tight hamstrings

MATCHING: Place the letter of the correct response in the space provided.

c	1. Annulus fibrosus	a.	Pain on the same side
l	2. Atlas	b.	Pain on the opposite side
m	3. Axis	c.	Outer covering of disc
f	4. Cauda equina	d.	Gelatin portion of disc
t	5. Cervical compression	e.	Motor stimulated by sensory neuron without involvement of the brain
s	6. Cervical distraction	f.	Nerve bundle that looks like a horse's tail
b	7. Contralateral	g.	Lateral rotational curve
q	8. Extruded disc	h.	Stress fracture of the pars interarticularis
a	9. Ipsilateral	i.	Bilateral fracture of the pars interarticularis
j	10. Kyphosis	j.	Excessive thoracic curve
k	11. Lordosis	k.	Excessive lumbar curve
o	12. Nucleus pulposus	l.	First cervical vertebra
p	13. Prolapsed disc	m.	Second cervical vertebra
e	14. Reflex	n.	Congenital defect in vertebral canal
g	15. Scoliosis	o.	Scheuermann's disease
r	16. Sequestrated disc	p.	Nucleus moves into fibers of the annulous fibrosus
n	17. Spina bifida occulta	q.	Eccentric nucleus moves into the spinal canal
i	18. Spondylolisthesis	r.	Eccentric nucleus separates from the disc and migrates
h	19. Spondylolysis	s.	Increased pain indicates soft tissue injury
o	20. Wedge fracture	t.	Increased pain indicates nerve root injury

ESSAY 1. Describe what measures can be taken to prevent low back pain in activities of daily living.

ESSAY 2. What actions should an individual perform to do a full scan examination of the spinal region?

ESSAY 3. Describe the danger signs that would indicate a possible cervical spine injury. If any of these are present, how would you manage the situation?

ESSAY 4. A runner is complaining of low back pain when sitting that increases when leaning forward. Pain is also present when running up hills and when running on concrete and has begun to radiate into the posterior leg. Using the HOPS format, assess this injury. What signs would indicate that this individual needs to be referred to a physician for follow-up care?

ESSAY 5. Discuss the purpose of flexion exercises versus extension exercises for the spine. Give examples of flexion and extension exercises that could be used in the beginning stages of a spinal rehabilitation program.

Chapter 15
Throat, Thorax, and Visceral Injuries

_d_ 1. Valves that prevent blood flow from the aorta and pulmonary arteries back into the ventricles are called:
a. Atrioventricular valves
b. Aorticpulmonary valves
c. Pulmonaryaortic valves
d. Semilunar valves

_d_ 2. The organ that cleanses the blood of foreign matter and stores excess red blood cells is the:
a. Kidney
b. Liver
c. Pancreas
d. Spleen

_c_ 3. The organ that secretes most of the digestive enzymes and the hormones insulin and glucogon is the:
a. Kidney
b. Liver
c. Pancreas
d. Spleen

_d_ 4. The muscle responsible for compression of the abdominal contents and aiding in forced expiration is the:
a. External oblique
b. Internal oblique
c. Rectus abdominus
d. Transverse abdominis

_d_ 5. A sharp pain or spasm in the chest wall on the lower right side that occurs during exertion is called a:
a. Liver contusion
b. Pneumothorax
c. Solar plexus stitch
d. Stitch in the side

_b_ 6. If an individual has a rib fracture, which of the following actions will not seriously increase pain?
a. Leaning away from the fracture site
b. Leaning toward the fracture site
c. Manual compression in an anteroposterior direction
d. Resisted trunk rotation and lateral flexion

_a_ 7. A direct blow to the anterolateral aspect of the thorax, a sudden twist, or falling on the ball can compress the rib cage, resulting in a:
a. Costochondral separation
b. Hemothorax
c. Kidney rupture
d. Solar plexus punch

_c_ 8. The most common intrathoracic injury in nonpenetrating chest trauma that may occur with forceful contact with another individual or in landing on a football is:
a. Hyperventilation
b. Pneumothorax
c. Pulmonary contusion
d. Tension pneumothorax

_c_ 9. An accumulation of air or gas in the pleural cavity that may occur spontaneously or as a result of trauma is called:
a. Hemothorax
b. Pneumonia
c. Pneumothorax
d. Thoracothetisitis

a 10. A condition in which the pleural cavity becomes filled with blood that has entered through an opening is called:
a. Hemothorax c. Thoracodorsalitis
b. Pneumothorax d. Traumatic asphyxia

c 11. An inherited connective tissue disorder affecting many organs, but commonly resulting in the dilation and weakening of the thoracic aorta is:
a. Cardiac tamponde c. Marfan's syndrome
b. Hypertrophic cardiomyopathy d. Mitral valve prolapse

a 12. A benign condition associated with physiologic alterations in the heart is called:
a. Athletic heart syndrome c. Hypertrophic cardiomyopathy
b. Cardiac tamponde d. Mitral valve prolapse

d 13. A protrusion of the abdominal viscera through a portion of the abdominal wall is called a/an:
a. Abdominal hydrocele c. Ganglion
b. Evisceration d. Hernia

d 14. The organ most often injured by blunt trauma that, if unrecognized, can lead to death is the:
a. Kidney c. Pancreas
b. Liver d. Spleen

b 15. Pain radiating to the left shoulder and arm could signal damage to:
a. Stomach c. Pancreas
b. Spleen d. Liver

a 16. Any athlete who receives a severe blow to the abdomen or back region should be instructed to check for:
a. Blood in the urine
b. Elevated blood pressure for several days afterwards
c. Elevated temperature for signs of internal infection
d. Visual acuity and headaches

d 17. Which of the following conditions can predispose an individual to injuries of the spleen?
a. Cirrhosis c. Hematuria
d. Eating right before competition d. Mononucleosis

b 18. A great danger with a ruptured spleen is its:
a. Ability to increase the incidence of constipation
b. Ability to splint itself and then produce delayed hemorrhage
c. High incidence of infection
d. Ineffectiveness in producing antibodies and red blood cells

a 19. When conducting the objective part of an injury assessment, which step should be completed first?
a. Auscultation c. Observation
b. Palpation d. Special tests

a 20. Pain referred to the posterior lumbar region radiating to the flanks and groin may indicate damage to the:
a. Kidney c. Pancreas
b. Liver d. Spleen

Matching: Place the letter of the correct response in the space provided.

c	1. Alveoli	a. Blood vessels between the lungs and heart
m	2. Arrhythmia	b. Blood vessels to the general body
d	3. Atria	c. Terminal air sacs of the bronchial tree
p	4. Auscultation	d. Superior heart chambers
n	5. Cardiac tamponade	e. Smooth muscle contractions move food through intestines
q	6. Celiac plexus	f. Paste-like substance into which food is churned
f	7. Chyme	g. Inflammation of liver caused by alcoholism
g	8. Cirrhosis	h. Inflammation of liver caused by viral infection
k	9. Cyclist's nipples	i. Spasmodic closure of the glottic aperture
l	10. Gynecomastia	j. Nipple irritation due to friction
r	11. Hematuria	k. Nipple irritation due to perspiration and windchill
h	12. Hepatitis	l. Excessive development of male mammary glands
i	13. Laryngospasm	m. Disturbance in heartbeat
t	14. McBurney's point	n. Compression of heart due to effusion of fluid into pericardium
e	15. Peristalsis	o. Nontraumatic, unexpected death
s	16. Proteinuria	p. Listening for sounds
a	17. Pulmonary circuit	q. Nerves that innervate abdominal region
j	18. Runner's nipples	r. Blood in urine
o	19. Sudden death	s. Protein in urine
b	20. Systemic circuit	t. Appendicitis pain

ESSAY 1. A basketball player was accidentally struck in the throat by an opponent's elbow and immediately dropped to the knees, coughing spasmodically. The individual has shortness of breath and is unable to speak. Using the HOPS format, assess this injury. What signs or symptoms would indicate that this individual needs to be transported immediately to a physician?

ESSAY 2. A wrestler was thrown to the mat, and his opponent fell on top of him. He is now complaining of pain on the anterior chest wall just lateral to the sternum. The localized sharp pain is followed by intermittent stabbing pain. Pain increases with lateral compression of the rib cage. Using the HOPS format, assess this injury. What possible condition may be present?

ESSAY 3. What signs and symptoms indicate an intra-abdominal injury? If one is suspected, what steps should be taken to manage the situation?

ESSAY 4. A gymnast is complaining of marked tenderness and muscle guarding along the abdominal wall during straight leg raising or hyperextension of the back. Using the HOPS format, assess this injury. What possible condition may be present?

ESSAY 5. A swimmer is complaining of an aching pain in the lower right quadrant of the abdomen. The pain has been present for 2 days but is getting worse. Using the HOPS format, assess this injury. What possible condition may be present?

Chapter 16
Conditions Related to the Reproductive System

_a_ 1. The organs that transport, protect, and nourish the gametes are called the:
a. Accessory sex organs
b. Mammary sex organs
c. Primary sex organs
d. Tertiary sex organs

_b_ 2. The hormone responsible for regulating the menstrual cycle and influencing the development of female physical sex characteristics is:
a. Androgen
b. Estrogen
c. Progesterone
d. Testosterone

_a_ 3. In managing a scrotal contusion, the first step is to:
a. Apply cold to the area
b. Call a doctor
c. Reduce testicular spasm
d. Apply compression

_b_ 4. Bikers may develop transient paresthesia of the penis, resulting from pressure to what nerve?
a. Penile nerve
b. Pudendal nerve
c. Scrotal nerve
d. Testicular nerve

_d_ 5. A severe blow to the testicular region that results in an excess of fluid accumulation is characteristic of a:
a. Scrotal contusion
b. Spermatic cord torsion
c. Testicular paramoritis
d. Traumatic hydrocele of the tunica vaginalis

_d_ 6. The first sign of testicular cancer is a(n):
a. Appearance of a bright red discoloration
b. Appearance of a cluster of swollen arteries
c. Appearance of a cluster of swollen veins with a dragging feeling in the scrotum
d. Slightly enlarged testicle and change in consistency

_a_ 7. Individuals with a(n) ____ are at a higher risk for developing testicular cancer.
a. Undescended testicle
b. Large testicles
c. Circumcised penis
d. None of the above

_b_ 8. Treatment for tinea cruris may include each of the following steps except:
a. Antifungal medication
b. Antibiotics
c. Keeping the groin area clean and dry
d. Wearing loose, absorbent clothing

_d_ 9. A visible painless ulcer or chancre at the site of entry is characteristic of what STD?
a. Chlamydia
b. Gonorrhea
c. Herpes
d. Syphilis

_b_ 10. Hepatitis primarily attacks what major organ, severely impairing function?
a. Brain
b. Liver
c. Pancreas
d. Spleen

d 11. All of the following are signs and symptoms of AIDS except:
   a. Dry cough
   b. Fatigue
   c. Shortness of breath
   d. Weight gain

a 12. Acquired immune deficiency syndrome can be transmitted in all of the following manners except:
   a. Casual contact with an individual with AIDS
   b. Passage from the mother to an unborn child through the placenta
   c. Receiving blood or other blood-product transfusions from an individual with AIDS
   d. Using infected hypodermic needles when injecting drugs

b 13. The syndrome identified by cramps, nausea, lower abdominal pain, and headache during menstruation is called:
   a. Amenorrhea
   b. Dysmenorrhea
   c. Menorrhagia
   d. Oligomenorrhea

c 14. When the menstrual cycle is normal but the cycle occurs more frequently, this condition may be present:
   a. Anovulation
   b. Exercise-associated amenorrhea
   c. Luteal phase deficiency
   d. Secondary amenorrhea

d 15. An individual with amenorrhea and decreased estrogen production is highly predisposed to:
   a. Anovulation
   a. Chondromalacia patellae
   c. Osteitis pubis
   d. Stress fractures

b 16. Oral contraceptives are designed to do each of the following except:
   a. Decrease the amount and duration of menstrual flow
   b. Prevent implantation of the fertilized ovum in the uterine lining
   c. Prohibit ovulation
   d. Reduce menstrual cramps

b 17. Side effects from taking oral contraceptive pills include all the following except:
   a. Breast tenderness
   b. Dehydration
   c. Increased risk of vaginitis
   d. Weight gain

c 18. During pregnancy, which hormones lead to joint laxity thereby increasing the risk for joint injuries?
   a. Estrogen and relaxin
   b. Estrogen and progesterone
   c. Progesterone and relaxin
   d. Relaxin and thyrotropin

b 19. Postural adaptations during pregnancy can lead to:
   a. Kyphosis
   b. Lordosis
   c. Scoliosis
   d. Upper spinal flexion

c 20. If a woman wants to continue exercising during pregnancy, she needs to do each of the following except:
   a. Consume extra carbohydrates
   b. Drink extra fluids
   c. Exercise in the supine position
   d. Strengthen the abdominals and hip extensors

MATCHING: Match the correct terms and place the answer in the space provided.

b	1. Accessory sex organs	a. Produce gametes
n	2. Amenorrhea	b. Transport, protect, and nourish gametes
f	3. Androgens	c. Phase when the vascular walls of the uterus are lost
l	4. Dysmenorrhea	d. Produce female secondary sex characteristics
d	5. Estrogens	e. Thickens the uterine wall for the fertilized ovum
i	6. Hematocele	f. Develop male genitals and secondary sex traits
g	7. Hydrocele	g. Tunica vaginalis swelling
c	8. Menses	h. Abnormal dilation of veins of the spermatic cord
m	9. Oligomenorrhea	i. Rapid accumulation of blood or fluid in scrotum
o	10. Osteopenia	j. Intense itching
a	11. Primary sex organs	k. Known to reverse the order of reproduction within the cells they infect
e	12. Progesterone	l. Painful menstruation
j	13. Pruritus	m. Infrequent menstrual cycle
k	14. Retroviruses	n. Cessation of menstruation
h	15. Varicocele	o. Decreased bone density

ESSAY 1. A rugby player was kicked in the groin by another player. He is on the pitch in a fetal position in extreme pain. What immediate concerns are present, and what signs and symptoms would indicate that a serious problem is present?

ESSAY 2. Describe different steps that can be taken to prevent tinea cruris.

ESSAY 3. What individuals are at risk for exposure to the hepatitis virus, and what measures can be taken in the athletic training room to prevent the spread of this disease?

ESSAY 4. What signs and symptoms would indicate that an individual may be infected by the HIV virus?

ESSAY 5. If a female sport participant wants to continue exercise during pregnancy, what guidelines should be suggested to allow continued exercise without compromising fetal development?

Chapter 17
Other Health Conditions Related to Sports

a 1. The single most important factor to prevent altitude sickness is:
a. Acclimatization
b. Arrive 2 days before competition
c. Eat a diet high in protein and salt
d. Inhale oxygen prior to competition

d 2. A colorless gas produced from burning coal or petroleum products that can be a potent bronchoconstrictor in asthmatics is:
a. Carbon monoxide
b. Ozone
c. Polycarbonate dioxide
d. Sulfur dioxide

b 3. Another name for the common cold is:
a. Bronchitis
b. Coryza
c. Pollinosis
d. Sinusitis

c 4. Which of the following is not a preventive measure for the common cold?
a. Avoid extreme fatigue
b. Avoid undue temperature changes by adjusting attire
c. Decrease fluid intake
d. Eat a balanced diet

d 5. An obstruction of the ostium due to local mucosal swelling, local insult, or mechanical obstruction is:
a. Bronchitis
b. Common cold
c. Pharyngitis
d. Sinusitis

a 6. Flu generally has an incubation period of:
a. 24 to 48 hours
b. 48 to 72 hours
c. 3 to 4 days
d. 4 to 6 days

c 7. An acute seasonal allergic condition that results from airborne pollens is called:
a. Bronchitis
b. Coryza
c. Hay fever
d. Pharyngitis

b 8. Hay fever may be relieved by:
a. Antifungal medications
b. Antihistamines
c. Aspirin
d. Nasal vasodilators

a 9. A condition resulting from infection and inhalants that can lead to inflammation of the mucosal lining of the tracheobronchial tree is called:
a. Bronchitis
b. Hay fever
c. Influenza
d. Rhinitis

b 10. Infectious mononucleosis is caused by which organism?
a. Adenoviruses
b. Epstein-Barr virus
c. Herpes simplex I
d. Herpes virus II

d 11. A common sign associated with bronchial asthma is:
a. Cyanosis
b. Lethargy
c. Prolonged rhinitis
d. Wheezing

a 12. Exercise-induced asthma typically develops how long after strenuous exercise begins?
a. 6 to 8 minutes
b. 15 to 20 minutes
c. 30 to 40 minutes
d. 1 hour

c 13. Which sport would produce the least chance of bronchospasm for an asthmatic athlete?
a. Cross-country running
b. Soccer
c. Swimming
d. Wrestling

d 14. Which of the following would not reduce the discomfort from diarrhea?
a. Drink boiled milk
b. Eat bland food
c. Eat a low-fiber diet 24 to 36 hours prior to practice
d. Reduce fluid intake before and during exercise

d 15. Which of the following is not a symptom of a diabetic coma?
a. Abdominal cramping
b. Dry mouth
c. Fruity smelling breath
d. Rapid onset

a 16. Which of the following is not a symptom of insulin shock?
a. Fruity smelling breath
b. Moist, pale skin
c. Physical weakness
d. Profuse sweating

c 17. A contagious disease that produces a skin rash on the face and body, rhinitis, photophobia, and fever is:
a. Chicken pox
b. German measles
c. Measles
d. Mumps

c 18. During a grand mal epileptic seizure, which of the following should not be done?
a. Remove furniture or obstructions from the area
b. Maintain airway
c. Force a tongue depressor in the mouth to prevent the tongue from occluding the airway
d. Turn athlete's head to the side so saliva and blood can drain

d 19. Anemia decreases all of the following except:
a. Efficiency at submaximal levels
b. Exercise time to exhaustion
c. Maximum aerobic capacity and anaerobic threshold
d. Predisposition to cirrhosis of the liver

a 20. Crisis symptoms for sickle cell anemia include all of the following except:
a. Hyperactivity
b. Painful hands and feet
c. Severe pain due to oxygen deprivation
d. Swollen and inflamed hands

MATCHING: Match the correct terms and place the answer in the space provided.

g	1. Asthma	a. Reduced oxygen to tissues
f	2. Bronchitis	b. Clear nasal discharge
h	3. Bronchospasm	c. Feeling out-of-sorts
p	4. Clonic state	d. The flu
k	5. Constipation	e. Seasonal allergic rhinitis
r	6. Coryza	f. Inflammation of tracheobronchial tree
m	7. Diabetes	g. Disease caused by constriction of the bronchial muscles
j	8. Diarrhea	h. Causes narrowing of the airway
t	9. Epilepsy	i. Inflammation of stomach or small intestine
i	10. Gastroenteritis	j. Loose or watery stools
e	11. Hay fever	k. Infrequent bowel movements
l	12. Hemorrhoids	l. Dilations of the veins in the rectal or anal area
n	13. Hyperglycemia	m. Disorder with near or absolute lack of insulin
o	14. Hypoglycemia	n. High levels of glucose in the blood
a	15. Hypoxia	o. Low levels of glucose in the blood
s	16. Infarcts	p. Repetitive muscle contraction and relaxation in rapid succession
d	17. Influenza	q. Steady rigid muscle contraction with no relaxation
c	18. Malaise	r. Common cold
b	19. Rhinorrhea	s. Clumping of cells that block blood vessels
q	20. Tonic state	t. Brain disorder with excessive discharges of electrical activity

ESSAY 1. What strategies can be implemented to prevent the onset of exercise-induced asthma?

ESSAY 2. What strategies can be implemented for a diabetic to prevent hypoglycemia or hyperglycemia during exercise?

ESSAY 3. Explain the three different types of seizures, and how you will manage the most severe type of an epileptic seizure.

ESSAY 4. In mid April, a lacrosse player suddenly begins to sneeze, has watery eyes, and a nasal discharge, and begins to feel dizzy. What condition is present, and how will you manage this situation?

ESSAY 5. A female gymnast is complaining of feeling tired at practice. She appears somewhat pale, and reports she has not had her period for the past 3 months. What conditions may have contributed to her fatigue? How will you handle this situation?